Changing Trends in Mental Health Care and Research in Ghana

Editors
Angela Ofori-Atta
Sammy Ohene

A READER OF THE DEPARTMENT OF PSYCHIATRY
UNIVERSITY OF GHANA MEDICAL SCHOOL

UNIVERSITY OF GHANA 65TH ANNIVERSARY READER PROJECT
CLINICAL SCIENCES SERIES NO 3

First published in Ghana 2014 for THE UNIVERSITY OF GHANA
by **Sub-Saharan Publishers**
P.O.Box 358
Legon-Accra
Ghana
Email: saharanp@africaonline.com.gh

P.O.Box LG 25
Legon- Accra
Ghana
Tel: +233-302-500381
website:http://www.ug.edu.gh

ISBN: 978-9988-8602-1-9

Cover page design: Samuel Adjei, KNUST 2013,

Contents

List of Tables

List of Figures

Foreword

The University of Ghana is celebrating sixty-five years of its founding this year. In all those years, lecturers and researchers of the university have contributed in quite significant ways to the development of thought and in the analyses of critical issues for Ghanaian and African societies. The celebration of the anniversary provides an appropriate opportunity for a reflection on the contributions that Legon academics have made to the intellectual development of Ghana and Africa. That is the aim of the University of Ghana Readers Project.

In the early years of the University, all the material that was used to teach students came largely from the United Kingdom and other parts of Europe. Most of the thinking in all disciplines was largely Eurocentric. The material that was used to teach students was mainly European, as indeed were many of the academics teaching the students. The norms and standards against which students were assessed were influenced largely by European values. The discussions that took place in seminar and lecture rooms were driven largely by what Africa could learn from Europe.

The 1960s saw a major 'revisionism' in African intellectual development as young African academics began to question received ideas against a backdrop of changing global attitudes in the wake of political independence. Much serious writing was done by African academics as their contribution to the search for new ways of organizing their societies. African intellectuals contributed to global debates in their own right and sometimes developed their own material for engaging with their students and the wider society.

Since the late 1970s universities in the region and their academics have struggled to make their voices heard in national and global debates. Against a new backdrop of economic stagnation and political disarray, many of the ideas for managing their economies and societies have come from outside. These ideas have often come with significant financial backing channelled through international organizations and governments. During the period, African governments saw themselves as having no reason to expect or ask for any intellectual contribution from their own academics. This was very much the case in Ghana.

The story is beginning to change in universities in many African countries. The University of Ghana Readers Project is an attempt to document the different ideas and debates that have influenced various disciplines over many years through collections of short essays and articles. They show the work of Legon academics and their collaborators in various disciplines as they have sought to introduce their research communities and students to new ideas. Our expectation is that this will mark a new beginning of solid engagement between Legon and other academics as they document their thoughts and contributions to the continuing search for new ideas to shape our world.

We gratefully acknowledge a generous grant from the Carnegie Corporation of New York that has made the publication of of this series of Readers possible.

Ernest Aryeetey
Vice-Chancellor, University of Ghana.
August 2013.

List of contributing authors and affiliated institutions

1. **Robert Acquah-Arhin**; Endwa M/A JHS. Ghana Education Service.
2. **J.K. Acquaye**; Professor, Department of Haematology, University of Ghana Medical School, Korle Bu Teaching Hospital.
3. **Akua A. Addae**; Assistant Lecturer, Department of Psychiatry, Universty of Ghana Medical School.
4. **Selassie Addom**; Medical Officer, Department of Psychiatry, Korle Bu Teaching Hospital.
5. **David Nana Adjei**; Statistician, School of Allied Health Sciences, Korle Bu Teaching Hospital.
6. **Dwomoa Adu**; Consultant Nephrologist, University of Ghana Medical School.
7. **Salma Yusuf Adusei**; Psychologist in training (MPhil), University of Ghana Medical School.
8. **Hannah Belle A. Anang**; Psychologist in training (MPhil), University of Ghana Medical School.
9. **G.A. Ankra-Badu**; Professor, Department of Haematology, University of Ghana Medical School, Korle Bu Teaching Hospital
10. **Adote Anum**; Neuropsychologist and Lecturer, Department of Psychology, University of Ghana.
11. **Ethel Akpene Atefoe**; Psychologist in training (MPhil), Universty of Ghana Medical School.
12. **Mary Ampomah**; Clinical Psychologist, Sickle Cell Clinic, Korle Bu Teaching Hospital.
13. **Timothy N. A. Archampong**; Lecturer; Dept of Medicine and Therapeutics, University of Ghana Medical School.

14. **J.B. Asare**; Adjunct Associate Professor of Psychiatry, SMHS University of Development Studies, Tamale. Retired Chief Psychiatrist, Ghana Health Service.
15. **Dzifa Attah**; Assistant Lecturer and Clinical Psychologist, Department of Psychiatry, University of Ghana Medical School.
16. **Dominic Atweam**; Health Information System Analyst, Information Monitoring Evaluation Dept, Policy Planning Monitoring and Evaluation Division., Ghana Health Service.
17. **Kwao Armah-Aloo**; Medical Director and Consultant Psychiatrist, Ankaful Psychiatric Hospital, Cape Coast.
18. **Seth Asafo**; Psychology Intern, Department of Psychiatry, University of Ghana Medical School.
19. **Patrick Boateng**; Medical Officer, Department of Psychiatry, Korle Bu Teaching Hospital.
20. **Vincent Boima**; physician specialist, nephrologist and lecturer, Department of Medicine, Korle Bu Teaching Hospital, Accra.
21. **Anna Dzadey**; Medical Director and Consultant Psychiatrist, Pantang Psychiatric Hospital.
22. **Ivy Ekem**; Senior Lecturer and Consultant Haematologist, Department of Haematology, University of Ghana Medical School.
23. **Vincent Ganu**; Medical Officer, Department of Medicine, University of Ghana Medical School, Korle Bu Teaching Hospital.
24. **Efe Ghanney**; Icahn School of Medicine, Mount Sinai, MD 2017.
25. **David Goldberg**; Institute of Psychiatry, King's College, London, U.K.
26. **Gabriel Ivbijaro**; Waltham Forest Community and Family Mental Health Services, The Wood Street Medical Centre, London, U.K.
27. **Helen Jack**; Yale University; New Haven, .CT. USA.
28. **Lucia Kolkiewicz**; East London NHIS Foundation Trust, London, U.K.

29. **Lily Kpobi;** Clinical Psychologist and Assistant Lecturer, Department of Psychiatry, University of Ghana Medical School.

30. **Crick Lund;** Director, Alan J Flisher Centre for Public Mental Health. Dept of Psychiatry and Mental Health, University of Cape Town, South Africa.

31. **C. Charles Mate-Kole;** PhD; Professor and Neuropsychologist, Departments of Psychology and Psychiatry, University of Ghana. Professor Emeritus,Central Connecticut State University,CT.USA.

32. **Michael Mate-Kole;** Associate Professor and Consultant Nephrologist, Department of Medicine, University of Ghana Medical School, Korle Bu Teaching Hospital.

33. **Anne Mensah-Kufuor;** Clinical Psychologist, Tetteh Quarshie Memorial Hospital, Ghana Health Service.

34. **The Mental Health and Poverty Project (MHaPP);** a Research Programme Consortium (RPC) funded by the UK Department for International Development (DfID)(RPC HD6 2005-2010) for the benefit of developing countries. The views expressed are not necessarily those of DfID. RPC members included Alan J. Flisher (Director) and Crick Lund (Co-ordinator) (University of Cape Town, Republic of South Africa (RSA)); Therese Agossou, Natalie Drew, Edwige Faydi and Michelle Funk (World Health Organization); Arvin Bhana (Human Sciences Research Council, RSA); Victor Doku (Kintampo Health Research Centre, Ghana); Andrew Green and Mayeh Omar (University of Leeds, UK); Fred Kigozi (Butabika Hospital, Uganda); Martin Knapp (University of London, UK); John Mayeya (Ministry of Health, Zambia); Eva N Mulutsi (Department of Health, RSA); Sheila Zaramba Ndyanabangi (Ministry of Health, Uganda); Angela Ofori-Atta (University of Ghana); Akwasi Osei (Ghana Health Service); and Inge Petersen (University of KwaZulu-Natal, RSA).

35. **Tolib Mirzoev;** Lecturer in International Health, Nuffield Centre for International Health & Development, Leeds Institute of Health Sciences, University of Leeds.

36. **Yasmin Mohammed**; Psychologist in Training (MPhil), Department of Psychiatry, University of Ghana Medical School.

37. **Seraphim Mork**; Graduate Student, Department of Psychology, Central Michigan University, USA.

38. **K. N. Nkrumah**; Senior Lecturer, Dept of Medicine and Therapeutics, University of Ghana Medical School.

39. **Angela Ofori-Atta**; Senior Lecturer and Clinical Psychologist, Department of Psychiatry, University of Ghana Medical School.

40. **Sammy Ohene**; Head, and Senior Lecturer, Department of Psychiatry, Consultant Psychiatrist, University of Ghana Medical School.

41. **Olive Okraku**; Graduate Student, Department of Psychology, University of Alberta, Canada.

42. **Judith Osae-Larbi**; Assistant Health Psychology Specialist Atlantis Healthcare, UK.

43. **Charlotte Osafo**; Consultant Nephrologist, University of Ghana Medical School.

44. **Akwasi Osei**; Chief Psychiatrist and Medical Director, Accra Psychiatric Hospital, Ghana Health Service.

45. **Ursula Read**; Career Development Fellow, MRC Social and Public Health Sciences Unit, Institute of Health and Well-Being, University of Glasgow.

46. **Joanna Salifu**; PhD Candidate, Department of Psychology, Stellenbosch University, South Africa,

47. **Abena Sarfo**; MPhil grauate student, Department of Psychology, University of Ghana Medical School.

48. **Araba Sefa-Dedeh**; Senior Lecturer and Clinical Psychologist, Department of Psychiatry, University of Ghana Medical School.

Section A:Mental Healthcare in Ghana

Chapter 1
Introduction

Angela Ofori-Atta and Sammy Ohene

This Reader is about the changing trends in mental healthcare and research in Ghana. It is a wonderful opportunity for us to showcase the work of the Department of Psychiatry (DOP) of the University of Ghana Medical School (UGMS), College of Health Sciences. The DOP is affiliated with the Korle Bu Teaching Hospital (KBTH), the Accra Psychiatric Hospital (APH) and Pantang Hospital for purposes of teaching, clinical practice, and research.

In the **Mental Healthcare in Ghana** section, we take you through the brief histories of mental healthcare in Ghana and of the DOP through the eyes of professionals who have lived this history. There is a reprint of a situation analysis of mental health services and legislation in 2005 which has been updated with respect to the Mental Health Law in order to capture the state of mental health services today. Following this introductory section are three main sections on **Conceptualization of Mental Illness, Mental Health practice in a Teaching Hospital Setting and Research in Psychiatry and Clinical Psychology.**

On **Conceptualization of Mental Illness,** we discuss depression, religion and illness, autism, substance use disorders and schizophrenia. The focus of the first two papers is on the non-medical, traditional conceptualization of illness (Ohene and Addom) and the impact of religious beliefs (Sefa-Dedeh). Salifu and Mate-Kole describe autism and give a good overview of the literature, while Asare and Addae discuss substance abuse and regulatory bodies in the Ghanaian setting. We conclude with a reprinted article of an overview of schizophrenia by Goldberg, Ivbijaro, Kolkiewicz and Ohene.

The Section on **Mental Health Practice in a Teaching Hospital Setting** emphasizes how these illnesses manifest, how people's lives are affected and what skill sets and resources are available for dealing with them. DOP has gradually expanded its scope of work to include Liaison

Psychiatry, which focuses on treating patients who are diagnosed with primarily physical or somatic complaints and who also report with underpinning mental health issues. In this section, Boateng, Ofori-Atta and Ohene describe the kind of referrals from KBTH and include two illustrative cases. The data show clearly that chronic physical illness has an impact on mental health and therefore treating patients with a bio-psychosocial model is absolutely necessary. Ampomah, Mate-Kole, Ofori- Atta et al. write on the neuropsychological difficulties in adult sickle cell patients. These tend to be overlooked as the more pressing and easily observable physical effects of sickle cell disease are attended to. The papers by Boima, Ganu, Adjei et al. on psychological problems in chronic renal disease patients, and by Archampong and Nkrumah on irritable bowel syndrome and related functional bowel disorders, both from the Department of Medicine, attest to the growing collaboration between the departments of Medicine and Psychiatry.

Collaboration between the Departments of Psychiatry and Child Health has generated services for mothers and their unwell infants and children. Anang, Adusei, Atefoe et al. and Osae-Larbi, Acquah-Arhin, Mork et al. contribute papers which describe group therapy with mothers of unwell neonates and play sessions with unwell children respectively. These interventions give support and relief from the stress of illness and may offer protective factors against post- natal depression and psychosis, and for children, perhaps prevent childhood depression, post-traumatic stress disorders and other forms of anxiety disorders. Asafo writes on breaking bad news to patients and helping physicians to accomplish this difficult and undesirable task with compassion and a sense of having held a patient's hand through a difficult part of the journey of illness. These three papers also stress the importance of psychosocial interventions in healthcare settings and point to the trend of things to come, namely, multi-disciplinary teams in the accomplishment of healthcare services for all. We believe that these interventions promote recovery from physical illness and we encourage research on the interaction between medicine and psychological therapies. We proudly note that the authors of the group therapy papers are trainee psychologists on practicum placement at the Department of Child-Health, while the paper on play groups was written by national service personnel assigned to the DOP. All papers in this section have reviews of the literature, and descriptions of the services offered. They are not research papers as such.

The final section is on research conducted in the Department of Psychiatry. The participants are medical students in Ofori-Atta, Okraku, and Mork et al.'s paper; children in school settings in Attah and Mate-Kole's paper; and health care professionals in Ofori-Attah and Jack's study on ethics. Finally, in Ofori-Atta, Mirzoev, Mensah-Kufuor et al.'s paper on the mental health information system, it is both health care professionals and the information system itself which are the subject of enquiry. Attah and Mate-Kole's paper was on Learning Disorders. With its focus on research, the Department has a large database still to be completely analysed, comprising work collected by various year groups of medical students in their senior clerkship in Psychiatry. For instance, the baseline information for the mental health information system was gathered by a group of senior clerkship students as they learned about the information system at the Accra Psychiatric and Pantang Hospitals in a qualitative study, while student interviews with healthcare professionals on ethical dilemmas formed the basis of the Jack et al. Ethics paper.

The interplay between teaching, clinical work and research has been truly rewarding for both faculty and students who also get the opportunity to present their findings at three annual conferences; the Annual Student Conference in Psychiatry, College of Health Sciences Annual Scientific Conference and the Psychiatry/Psychology Joint Conferences each year.

Although the Department of Psychiatry is relatively small, with three full time senior lecturers, an adjunct professor of psychology, two research officers, two assistant lecturers, and clinical support from three senior house officers and a senior medical officer, its output in research, in teaching and in clinical services in the past five years has been noteworthy. We hope you enjoy this array of readings in mental health in Ghana.

Chapter 2
Overview of Mental Health Care in Ghana

Lily Kpobi, Akwasi Osei and Araba Sefa-Dedeh

Pre-Colonial Psychiatric Care & Treatment

Before the advent of colonial rule in Ghana, all illnesses, including mental illnesses, were treated by local spiritual/traditional healers (Ewusi-Mensah, 2001). Most illnesses were attributed to external spiritual forces and were therefore treated with a supernatural focus for healing with the aid of plants, earth, and various other objects (Harding, 1975). Illness was therefore seen as an imbalance between the physical and spiritual world. With this belief, traditional healers were often more focused on identifying the cause of the illness, rather than the effects that the treatment methods had on the person physically, believing that the physical body would be restored to health when the spiritual imbalances were restored (Harding, 1975).

Treatment for illness usually included a relative or close family member learning from the healer and continuing care at home. This greatly facilitated their re-entry into the community and reduced the risk of family abandonment (Burler, 1997).

Mental Healthcare in Colonial Times

With the dawn of colonialism however, traditional healing practices were considered primitive and evil and were subsequently suppressed (Harding, 1975). Western beliefs and values were perpetuated and the mentally ill (called "lunatics" at the time) were often segregated and detained in prisons. In 1888 however, then-Governor Sir Edward Griffiths signed a Legislative Instrument to provide custody of people with mental illness to the state. He ordered the conversion of the old High Court of Victoriaborg (modern day Accra Central) into a "lunatic asylum" for the detention of mentally ill people. The staff at the asylum consisted of wardens who looked after the inmates. There were 11 attendants, a matron and a gatekeeper who monitored the

Patients were taken through activities such as psycho-education on the patients' drugs, current affairs and drama or role playing. Patients in this programme appeared to recover faster but relapsed when the programme was stopped. It was therefore decided to extend the programme into actual communities, in the belief that social conditions contributed to outcomes in psychiatric illness.

The Community Psychiatric Nursing programme was integrated into primary healthcare from 1986 and has served as the first point of contact for psychiatric patients in many districts across the country. Over 300 nurses have been deployed in all 10 regions of Ghana and work daily to reach both new and already diagnosed mentally ill people (Asare, 2003; Doku, Ofori-Atta, Akpalu et al., 2008). Community psychiatric nurses therefore regularly follow up discharged patients and educate their families and communities on mental illness, as well as continued care of the patient; they also work to create awareness and promote mental health within communities (Asare, 2003).

In addition to community psychiatric nursing care, patients also have access to social welfare officers who help with their social needs such as making arrangements for finances, housing, and mediating with children and spouses when needed. This is primarily to aid in the patient's recovery without the added pressures of their social lives plaguing them. See Figure 2 on page 10 for distribution of psychiatric nurses around the country.

Mental Health Legislation in Ghana

The Lunatic Asylum Ordinance Cap 79 of 1888 remained in existence until 1972 when NRC Decree 30 ("the Mental Health Act 1972") was enacted. This decree was primarily focused on providing institutional care of patients. It was an improvement on the 1888 ordinance, in terms of voluntary treatment and care. Despite attempts in 1996 to amend the decree, it remained the major legislation for mental health care in Ghana for many decades.

Since 2006 however, extensive work was done to introduce a Mental Health Bill to replace the 1972 Act. Despite its improvement

Fig 2.2: Distribution of psychiatric nurses per 100,000 people (Jack, 2011)

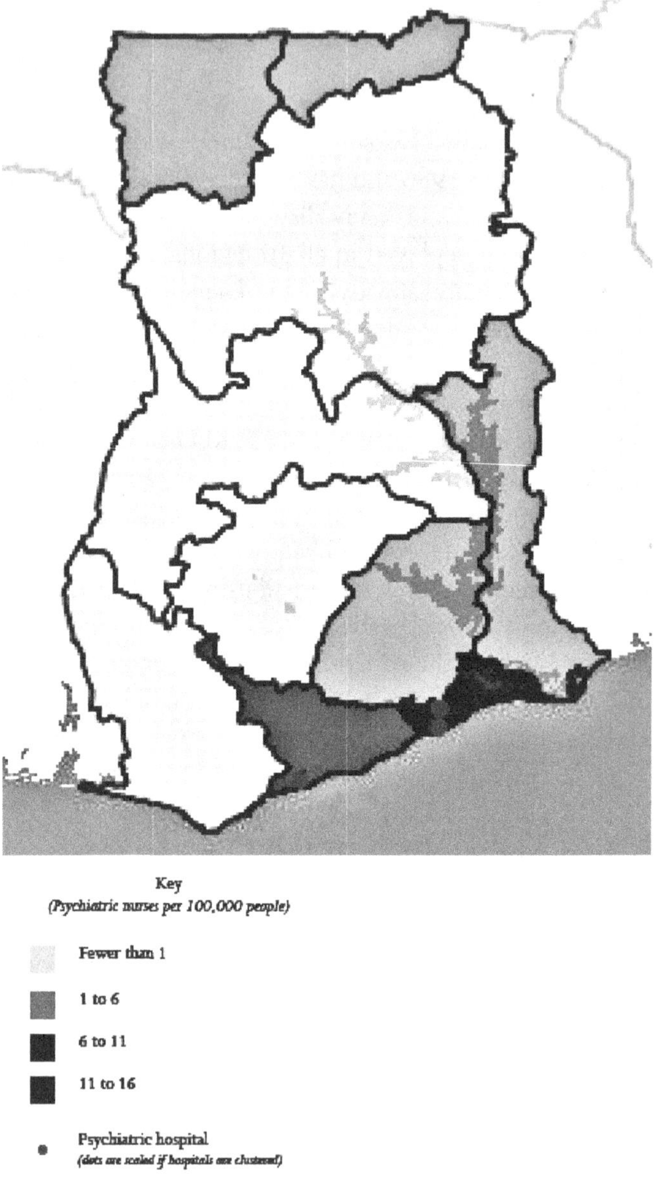

on the 1888 Ordinance, the 1972 Act was by then outdated and did not meet best practice standards including protection and improvement of the wellbeing of people living with mental illness (Ofori-Atta, Read & Lund, 2010).

In March 2012, the Parliament of Ghana successfully passed the new Mental Health Bill into law. The new law, (Act 846, 2012), attempts through legislation to bridge the gap between mental health needs and services in the country, and also focuses on the human rights of mentally ill people. The new law thus adopts a human rights-based approach to treatment of mental illness. It discourages discrimination and inhumane treatment, and seeks to provide equal opportunities for mentally ill people. It also provides for decentralized services with tertiary and regional level care being emphasized, and the integration of mental health care into Primary Health Care. Further, it makes provision for community-based mental health care to be properly established across the country.

Under the new law, mental health care financing is required as a priority in the health sector. This should translate into improvements of not only services, but also better human resources management of mental healthcare professionals. With approximately 18 psychiatrists in active practice, plus 30 practicing psychologists, the field of mental health care needs a serious influx of professionals. This new law provides for the employment of more workers to aid in service delivery. In the second quarter of 2013, the Ghana Health Service hired its first group of clinical psychologists and placed one in each regional hospital; a good sign of things to come.

Conclusion

From the pre-colonial period through colonial times to the post-independence period, mental healthcare in Ghana as a priority has generally been low. Often, facilities and human resources are inadequate and therefore tend to fall short of optimal standards. With the passing of the new Mental Health Law, the future of mental healthcare in Ghana is looking bright. Exciting times lie ahead as service provision is scaled up and a future is envisioned where the mentally ill have equal opportunities and where first-class care of the mentally ill is available everywhere.

References

Asare, J.B. (2003). *Mental Health Profile (Ghana).* Retrieved from WHO Africa Regional office website, http://www.afro.who.int/index.php.

Burler, B. (1997). The Treatment of Psychiatric Illness in Ghana. *African-Diaspora, 50.* Retrieved from http://digitalcollections.sit.edu/african_african_diaspora_isp/50.

Doku, V., Ofori-Atta, A., Akpalu, B. et al. (2008). A situation analysis of mental health policy development and implementation in Ghana. Mental Health and Poverty Country Report on Ghana. http://workhorse.pry.uct.ac.za:8080/MHAPP.

Ewusi-Mensah, I. (2001). Post-colonial Psychiatric Care in Ghana. *Psychiatric Bulletin*, *25*, 228 – 229.

Forster, E.B. (1962). A Historical Survey of Psychiatric Practice in Ghana. *Ghana Medical Journal.1 (1),* 25 – 29.

Harding, T.W. (1975). Traditional Healing Methods for Mental Disorders. *WHO Chronicle, 31,* 436 – 440.

Historical Background. (n.d.). Retrieved March, 2013 from Accra Psychiatric Hospital website, www.accrapsychiatrichospital.org

Jack, H. (2011). *"There is no motivation here": Exploring how to expand mental health care services in Ghana by addressing the needs of the workforce.* Yale University (Unpublished Thesis)

Ministry of Health. (1998). *The Centenary of the Accra Psychiatric Hospital: 1888 – 1988.* Ghana: Government Publications.

Ofori-Atta, A., Read, U.M., & Lund, C., and the MHaPP Research Programme Consortium (2010). A situation analysis of mental health services and legislation in Ghana: challenges for transformation. *African Journal of Psychiatry.* 13:99-108.

Osei, A. (2006, June 1). Accra Psychiatric Hospital is 100. *The Daily Graphic Newspaper,* p.9.

Twumasi, P. (1975). Medical Systems in Ghana: A Study in Medical Sociology. Accra: Ghana Publishing..

Chapter 3
History of the Department of Psychiatry
Araba Sefa–Dedeh

A history of the Department of Psychiatry appropriately starts with F.B. Forster; the first African psychiatrist south of the Sahara. Forster started working in Ghana in 1951 and was involved in the planning and establishment of the Medical School in 1962. He ensured the integration of psychiatry into the curriculum of the Medical School and became the first Head of Department. Until 1970, he was both Head of Department and Head of the Accra Psychiatric Hospital. It was this dual role that led to the siting of the Department at the Accra Psychiatric hospital. After 1970, Forster gave up headship of the hospital. He continued to serve as Head of Department till 1980 and was instrumental in the training of other psychiatrists who became his colleagues and took over from him.

C.C. Adomakoh, who had worked with Forster since 1970, became Head in 1980 and continued till 1987. He shepherded the department through some of the most difficult economic times in the department's history. Another colleague he served with at the time was J.J. Lamptey who had joined the department in October of 1971.

In 1971, S. Danquah joined the department as its first clinical psychologist. He was followed by Zonke Majodina from South Africa in 1973, Araba Sefa-Dedeh in 1980, Angela Ofori-Atta in 1992 and recently, C. Mate-Kole, a neuropsychologist, in 2009. In conjunction with other clinical psychologists who have served the department as researchers and tutors, they have been instrumental in establishing a vibrant unit that collaborates effectively with psychiatrists in a team approach which benefits students and patients and stimulates research.

S.N.A. Turkson became Head of Department in 1987. During his tenure, he mentored a number of young medical officers and he was instrumental in their training as psychiatrists. Most of them work outside Ghana, but some volunteer their services during the senior clerkship. Isaac Ewusi-Mensah joined the department in 1995. Sammy K. Ohene, who became Head of Department in 2005, joined the department in 1990. The last psychiatrist to have joined the department is Joel Abayomi Fashola in 2006. Despite the fact that there have never been more than three psychiatrists in full-time service in the department, their sacrificial work has ensured effective teaching for students and clinical services for numerous patients.

Two research officers, A. Nortey Dua and Kwame Asante joined the department in 1989. They had been clinical psychology students in the department and continued on after graduation. In addition to his official designation, Nortey Dua has been an integral part of the department's teaching programme over the years.

In recent times the department has employed tutors to help with the clinical training of its students. Olive O. Okraku and Alphonsus Tenteh did so in 2006, Dzifa Attah and Akua Afriyea Addae in 2010. In 2011, Edwin Boakye Yiadom was recruited as a research assistant to augment research efforts in the department.

Part-Time Lecturers

Despite the hard work of its teaching staff, the department could not have sustained its teaching without the help of part-time faculty. F. K. Amarquaye and C.C. Adomakoh helped Forster. J. B. Asare, G. A. Abbey, F. Atta Johnson, A. Osei, V. Doku and Dinah Baah-Odoom have all been very helpful in keeping the department's teaching schedule on course. In recent times help has come from faculty outside Ghana. Most are Ghanaians working in the UK, USA, and Canada but there are a few non-Ghanaian volunteers as well. Some of them are on a programme started by Doku but some personally bear the cost of their transportation and board to come and teach especially during the senior clerkship. Albert Gyimah from Canada and others from the USA have consistently helped. They include; Thad Ulzen, Gina Addae, Ama Addo, Ebenezer Okyere, Thomas Holdbrook, M. Murad, Bakht, Daniel Gboloo-Teye, Asamoah, Obodai Sai, Ocansey and Akanzua.

Teaching Programmes

The department's teaching programmes have changed over the years and it has kept abreast with modern developments in mental health education and care. At first, psychiatry was taught only during the junior and senior clerkships. Now students are tutored in introductory psychology in year two and medical psychology in year five. Apart from being introduced to the basics of diagnosis and clinical care in psychiatry during the senior clerkship, students research mental health problems, collect data, and present their findings in a conference. Psychiatry is examined in the final-year medical examination as part of Medicine, a practice that took some years and persuasion to establish.

The department jointly teaches and supervises a clinical practicum for MPhil clinical psychology students. It is also very much involved in the administration, teaching and examination of the Fellowship programmes of the Ghana College of Physicians and Surgeons and the West African College of Physicians (WACP). Forster was the second president of the WACP. He and Adomakoh started training residents in the 1970s even before the colleges were established. In 2012, Ohene completed his term as the chief examiner in psychiatry for the WACP.

Research

From the beginning of its establishment, the department has done research in its local setting. Forster pioneered research into schizophrenia and depression in Ghana. Adomakoh was interested in alcohol and substance abuse in Ghana. Sefa-Dedeh is researching religion and mental health and has worked with Ofori-Atta and Nortey Dua on the impact of health on cognition in children and in establishing local norms for psychological tests. Sefa-Dedeh, Ofori-Atta and Ohene set up mental health services in the Upper West Region in the 1990s and researched the use of alcohol in the rural communities of that region. Ofori-Atta worked on the Mental Health and Poverty Project in four African countries, a research consortium funded by Department for International Development, U.K. She also worked on high-level advocacy in conjunction with Yale University's Global Health Leadership Institute and the South Essex Partnership Trust. She is currently working on joining forces with prayer camps to introduce medication to patients with severe mental illness. Ohene is researching depression and student mental health in addition to epilepsy in Ghana. Turkson researched depression in women in Ghana and the quality of referrals for mental health care from general hospitals with Dua. Recent departmental interests include sexual abuse and mental health, drug abuse and dependence and the interface between general health and mental health services. It is also in discussion with psychiatrists at Harvard University and Massachusetts General Hospital for collaboration on mutual interests, and similarly with the South Essex Partnership Trust in the United Kingdom.

Facilities

The Department of Psychiatry was sited at the Accra Psychiatric Hospital from its inception till 2003 when it relocated to Korle Bu to be physically part of the rest of the Medical School. The move has led to a greater interaction and collaboration with other departments of the school and the hospital itself. At present, clinical psychology students do practicum in Child Health, Haematology, Fevers Unit, Sickle Cell Clinic, Plastic Surgery, Renal Unit, and Burns as well as the Addictions Services Unit. The department is a Sub Budget Management Center (BMC) of the Korle Bu Teaching Hospital and has been assigned a ward which is to be set up as a model for in-patient psychiatric care in a teaching hospital.

We are looking forward to even greater collaboration with the Hospital and other departments of the Medical School.

Chapter 4

An Updated Situation Analysis of Mental Health Services and Legislation in Ghana: Challenges for Transformation

A. Ofori-Atta, U.M. Read, C. Lund, and the MHaPP Research Programme Consortium[1]

Introduction

Mental health care is often one of the lowest health priorities for low-income countries (World Health Organisation WHO 2001) and Ghana is no exception. In common with many low-income post-colonial countries in Africa, Ghana has not developed the infrastructure and public services, including mental health care, to keep pace with population expansion. The population of Ghana has more than doubled since independence in 1957 and currently stands at approximately 25 million (Ghana Demographic & Health Survey; 2003, 2005) with a consequent growth in the numbers of people suffering from mental disorders. Research has revealed the extent to which mental health care in many low- and middle-income countries is consistently under-resourced.(Jacob, Sharan, Mirza, et al 2007; Kohn, Saxena, Levav, Saraceno, 2004; Saxena, Thornicroft, Knapp & Whiteford, 2007)

In the relative absence of community care, institutionalised care remains the norm for many of those with mental health problems in low-income countries (Saxena et al., 2007). Indeed, in countries such as Ghana, many of those in need of treatment do not reach psychiatric services at all, but seek the care of informal community mental health services (WHO, 2003) such as traditional and faith healers as well as family members who offer a varying quality of service and level of efficacy. In addition, there is increasing evidence from developing countries that mental illness is strongly associated with poverty (Patel, 2001; Patel & Kleinman, 2003; Saraceno, Levav & Kohn, 2005).

Despite some significant economic growth in recent years, Ghana is classified as a low-income country with 28.5 percent of the population living in poverty, and 18.2 percent living in extreme poverty, especially in rural areas (Government of Ghana, 2007). Yet there is a growing body of research demonstrating innovative, cost-effective interventions for mental disorders such as schizophrenia and depression in low-income African countries (Wiley-Exley, 2007; Patel, Araya, Chatterjee, et al., 2007; Siskind, Bolton & Kim, 2007).

Among these are agricultural rehabilitation villages in Tanzania (Kilonzo and Simmons,1998), family involvement in hospital care in Senegal (Diop & Dores, 1976; Franklin, Sarr, Gueye et al., 1996), group therapy for the treatment of depression in Uganda (Bolton,Bass, Neugebauer, et al., 2003), and collaborations with traditional healers in northern Ghana (Montia, 2008). In Africa therefore, as in other regions of the world, the deficit is not in the evidence for interventions to address mental health problems, but in the resources and political will that can make these interventions available to those who need them.

Ghana currently stands in a relatively unique position within the African continent to respond to this challenge. In spite of its low-income status, the country has one of the highest literacy rates (57.9 percent) within West Africa (United Nations Development Programme, 2005), is considered a relatively stable and peaceful democracy, with relatively good standards of governance, and has a strong and diverse civil society. Gaining independence as early as 1957, it was also one of the pioneers of primary health care in the region (Twumasi, 1974) and initiated attempts to develop mental health care in the first years of independence with the establishment of new psychiatric hospitals and later the introduction of clinical psychology, occupational therapy and community psychiatric nursing. Today, despite the shortage of specialist psychiatric personnel, Ghana remains relatively well-resourced for mental health care in comparison to other countries in the region (Jacob, Sharan, Mirza, et al., 2007).

There have been several attempts to respond to the call to develop mental health provision in primary care and to provide community-based mental health services. The training of community psychiatric nurses was instituted in 1976 when these nurses were posted to approximately half the districts in the country. Between 1994 and 1998 primary health care and development workers in the Upper West Region of Ghana were trained in mental health care, integrating mental health into primary care (Sefa-Dedeh, Ofori-Atta, Ohene et al., 2006). Similarly, in 1998 the World Health Organisation (WHO) *Nations for Mental Health Project* trained health volunteers to provide community support to patients with mental disorders (Asare, 2003; WHO, 2002).

Despite these innovations, a comprehensive situation analysis of the mental health system in Ghana has not yet been undertaken. This paper presents the results of a situation analysis of the current status of mental health policy and services in Ghana which was conducted as part of the first phase of the Mental Health and Poverty Project (MHaPP). The MHaPP, which was conducted in four African countries; Ghana, South Africa, Uganda and Zambia, investigated the policy level-interventions required to break the vicious cycle of poverty and mental ill-health, in order to generate lessons for a range of low- and middle-income countries (Flisher, Lund, Funk, et al., 2007). Based on the findings of the situation analysis, the paper presents proposals for transforming mental health care in Ghana to provide for the majority of those in need and to protect the human rights of patients and their families in a way which is culturally responsive and cost-effective.

Methods

The WHO Assessment Instrument for Mental Health Systems Version 2.2 (WHO AIMS, 2005) was completed by the researchers with the aid of 48 key stakeholders in health and mental healthcare in order to provide an overview of mental health policy and services. Data for the WHO-AIMS were collected for the index year of 2005.

Documentary analysis of mental health legislation was conducted utilising the WHO Checklist for Mental Health Legislation (WHO 2005), which is designed to assess the content and development of mental health legislation, according to a number of criteria. The checklist was completed by a team consisting of a clinical psychologist, a psychiatrist, a research officer, the national coordinator of community psychiatric nurses (CPNs), and the deputy director of nursing services at the Accra Psychiatric Hospital. Documents evaluated included: the 1972 Mental Health Decree (National Redemption Council Ghana, 1972) and the 2006 draft Mental Health Bill (GOG 2006).

Eighty-one interviews and seven focus group discussions were held with policy makers, health professionals, healers, users of psychiatric services, teachers, police officers, academics, and religious and traditional leaders drawn from five of the ten regions in Ghana. The interviews and focus group discussions were conducted with 122 respondents, who were purposively sampled from among the major stakeholders in mental health at the national, regional and district levels.

Semi-structured interview guides were tailored according to the specific individual being interviewed. Topics covered included general policy making process in Ghana, the process of mental health policy and legislation development, the role of stakeholders in mental health policy and legislation development, the content of the current mental health policy and legislation, and the implementation of mental health policy and legislation at the national and regional levels. Thirty-five interviews were held at the national level, and 23 at the regional level. One focus group discussion was held at the national level.

Interviews were digitally recorded with participants' consent and transcribed verbatim. Interviews in local Ghanaian language (Twi) were first transcribed and then translated into English by staff of the Bureau of Ghana Languages. All transcripts were entered into Nvivo 7 which was used for coding and analysis. A framework analysis approach was adopted (Ritchie & Spencer, 1994) in which certain themes were agreed upon by investigators from all four study countries based on the objectives of the study. From these objectives, sub-themes were suggested by country partners, and reviewed by all partners through a process of iteration, until a single framework was agreed upon that could be used by all four study countries. Where specific themes emerged from the interviews that were not included in the generic cross-country framework, these were added to the coding frame, to adapt the analysis to issues specific to Ghana. Transcripts were coded on the basis of these themes, with additional themes added to the coding framework as determined by the data. Interviews were coded independently for 10 percent of randomly sampled interviews to ensure inter-rater reliability. Inter-rater reliability was always above 90 percent.

Ethical approval was granted by the Ghana Health Service Ethics Committee and the Institutional Ethics Board at Kintampo Health Research Centre. Information sheets containing essential information about the study and the implications of participation were given to all participants. Participants who were unable to read had a witness read the information sheet and consent form to them in Twi. Participants were requested to sign a consent form to indicate their willingness to participate in the study. Those participants who were unable to write were requested to provide a thumb print in lieu of a signature in the presence of a witness. The names and other identifying features of the respondents were removed from the transcripts in order to ensure confidentiality.

Results

Policy, governance and organisational structure

Policy is formulated at the ministerial level in the Ministry of Health (MOH), and implemented through the Ghana Health Service (GHS). The Mental Health Unit, which had oversight of mental health services, was placed under GHS Institutional Care Division (see Figure 4.1). The Mental Health Unit acted as the national mental health authority, advising the government on mental health policies and legislation, and providing monitoring and quality assessment of mental health services. The Unit had oversight of the three government psychiatric hospitals, the psychiatric wings of the five regional hospitals, community mental health services, and private psychiatric facilities. Traditional and faith healers were also supposed to be under the supervision of the unit. However, in practice, there was little oversight (see Figure 4.1). These functions were supposed to be taken over by the Mental Health Authority when it is set up under the new Mental Health Law.

Fig 4.1: Organisation of mental health services in Ghana

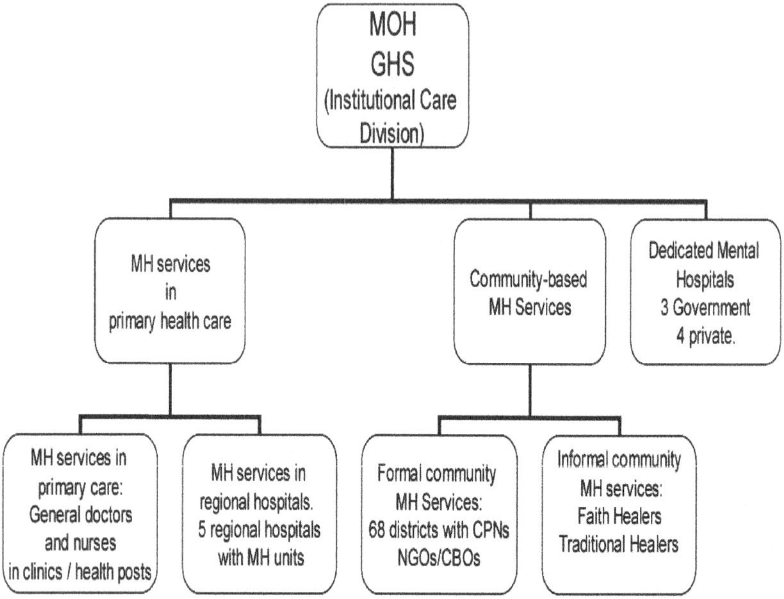

Financing of Mental Health Services

It was reported that approximately 6.2 percent of the health care budget of the Ministry of Health was dedicated to mental health in 2005. The results of interviews with mental health professionals and Ministry of Finance officials indicated that due to the policy of de-centralisation, funding was disbursed to Budget Management Centres at the regional and district levels, some of which may have been allocated to mental health. However there were no figures available on mental health expenditure at the district level.

The majority of the budget for mental health (nearly 80 percent) was allocated for the maintenance of the three psychiatric hospitals. Despite this, funding for the psychiatric hospitals was described by one psychiatric nurse as "woefully inadequate". Participants reported that funds were quickly absorbed in meeting the basic needs of patients, and the psychiatric hospitals often run out of sufficient funds to feed patients. Therefore little of the budget was available for psychosocial and rehabilitative interventions.

The National Health Insurance Scheme (NHIS) does not cover psychiatric services because by policy, treatment for mental disorders is provided free of charge at the government psychiatric hospitals and through community psychiatric nurses. However, if these are not accessible, or medication runs out, as does occur, then patients have to purchase these privately without recourse to a refund. Many psychiatric patients who do not have health insurance are not covered for treatment of co-morbid physical conditions.

Mental health services

Inpatient care

There are three government psychiatric hospitals in Ghana providing 7.04 beds per 100,000 population. Accra and Pantang psychiatric hospitals are located in Accra, and Ankaful Psychiatric Hospital is in the Central Region. In 2005, there were four private psychiatric institutions which provided outpatient clinics and inpatient care. Two were located close to Accra and two near the second largest city of Kumasi. There were psychiatric inpatient units in 5 of the 10 regional general hospitals in the country providing a total of 77 beds (0.33 beds per 100,000 population), with the number of beds per unit ranging from 10 to 22. The ratio of psychiatric beds in the mental hospitals in or around Accra, the capital, to the total number of beds in mental hospitals in the rest of the country was 6.28 to 1, indicating a concentration of inpatient resources in urban areas.

There were 6,605 admissions to the three state psychiatric hospitals in 2005. Approximately 50 percent of these were female. It is likely that this number included repeat admissions due to the failure to capture unique patient identifiers in the health information system. The state psychiatric hospitals were chronically overcrowded by as much as a third more patients than beds.

Inpatient stays were frequently lengthy, which exacerbated the pressure on hospital beds (Table 4.1). According to stakeholders, one of the reasons for such long admissions was the stigma associated with mental disorders, which resulted in relatives or caregivers abandoning the person in hospital. Secondly, in hospital patients receive free board and lodging, as well as treatment. This was an attractive benefit for both the patient and the family, particularly those with limited financial means. In addition, due to the absence of secure hospitals and the inefficiency of the legal system, some offenders who had been ordered by the courts to be admitted for a psychiatric assessment could remain in the psychiatric hospitals for many months or abscond to avoid justice.

Table 4.1: Number of beds and average length of inpatient admission to psychiatric hospitals

Hospital	Bed capacity	Average length of hospital admission	Number of long stay patients*
Ankaful	250	82.2 days	Not available
Pantang	500	285 days	205
Accra	800	Not available	520

**patients who had recovered but remain in hospital*

Psychotic disorders were the most frequent inpatient diagnosis in the psychiatric hospitals, followed by substance use disorders and mood disorders (Table 4.2). Neurotic disorders were rarely diagnosed and recorded. There were also many cases with unspecified diagnoses. There are difficulties interpreting the data as diagnosis is frequently not standardised, according to several stakeholders who were interviewed.

Table 4.2: Inpatient diagnoses at psychiatric hospitals in Ghana, 2005

Diagnosis	Accra	Pantang	Ankaful	Total	%
Mental and behavioural disorders due to psycho-active substance use (F10- F19)	808	338	362	1508	22.8
Schizophrenia, schizotypal, and delusional disorders (F20-F29)	1442	516	511	2469	37.4
Mood, affective disorders (F30-39)	605	138	510	1253	19.0
Neurotic, stress-related and somatoform disorders (F40-F48)	0	0	0	NR	
Disorders of adult person-ality and behaviour (F60-F69)	0	0	0	NR	
Others*	1232	86	57	1375	20.8
Total				6605	100

**includes epilepsy, dementia, other organic disorders, and unspecified*
NR not recorded

(Outpatient care)

A total of 86,003 cases were attended to at the outpatient departments of the three psychiatric hospitals in 2005 (Table 4.3). There is likely to be some overlap in these statistics since some patients attended more than one psychiatric hospital.

Table 4.3: Outpatient attendance by gender at psychiatric hospitals in Ghana, 2005

Hospital	Male	Female	Total
Accra	20,462	23,682	44,211
Pantang	6,922	5,963	12,885
Ankaful	N/A	N/A	28,907
Total	N/A	N/A	86,003

(N/A = not available)

Sub-Specialist Services

There were no dedicated outpatient facilities for child and adolescent mental health in Ghana. A total of 2,578 patients under the age of 19 years were seen at all three hospitals. There were 45 dedicated inpatient beds for children and adolescents in the psychiatric hospitals, representing 4 percent of the total. There were 10 residential facilities for children under 17 with intellectual disabilities, one in each of the regions. In addition, a non-governmental organisation (NGO) provided residential care and rehabilitation in the Brong Ahafo Region for children with intellectual disabilities. There was also a private school for children with intellectual disabilities in Accra. There were dedicated beds for older people at the Accra Psychiatric Hospital. However, there was no specialised mental health service for older people, or people with dementia.

In Accra Psychiatric Hospital there was a dedicated forensic ward with 15 beds and more than 300 patients. However this ward was not used solely by forensic patients. In Pantang hospital in 2005, there were 88 forensic patients. There were two private residential facilities for people with substance abuse disorders and one private hospital in Accra had a detoxification unit.

Rehabilitation, residential and day services

There were very few rehabilitation and day services for people with mental disorders. Those which existed were largely run by NGOs and faith-based organisations. There were 15 beds in an inpatient rehabilitation facility which formed part of Ankaful Psychiatric Hospital and six community residential facilities run by voluntary and church organisations which provided drug rehabilitation. Cheshire Home in Kumasi provided residential rehabilitation and vocational training for up to 55 adults with mental disorders. The NGOs BasicNeeds and Christian Blind Mission had established three community-based rehabilitation projects for people with mental disorders in the north of Ghana. Since 2010, Pantang Hospital had a residential addiction rehabilitation programme.

There were three known day-treatment facilities in Ghana run by NGOs or church organisations. The Damien Centre at Takoradi in the southwest of the country was run by the Catholic church. Two drop-in facilities for vagrants were provided in Tamale in the Northern Region based on the Club House model: Tsi-sampa run by Basic Needs, and Shekina, run by a private practitioner. There were no day-treatment facilities run by GHS.

Mental health in primary health care

Doctors provide primary mental health care through the outpatient departments of the hospitals. Most government clinics in the sub-districts do not employ doctors, but are staffed by medical assistants or nurses, or by personnel with lower levels of training such as community health workers or community midwives. Medical assistants provide assessment, diagnosis and treatment, including prescribing and administering medication, and effectively work in a physician assistant role. There are no specialist doctors in mental health in primary health care clinics in Ghana. In spite of this, there are assessment and treatment protocols in most of these clinics which include guidance on the treatment of the major psychiatric conditions including schizophrenia and depression (Ghana Health Service, 2004).

Table 4.4: Outpatient psychiatric service utilisation per region, 2005

Disorder	WR	CR	GAR	VR	ER	ASH	BAR	NR	UER	UWR	Total
Epilepsy	868	200	929	911	581	1,239	737	733	1,005	458	7,661
Acute Psychosis	194	123	1,607	1,612	755	1,044	1,065	221	645	184	7,450
Neurosis	288	276	524	304	431	4,101	660	108	332	103	7,127
Substance Abuse	443	139	739	269	482	1,452	261	84	333	119	4,321
Total new cases	**1,793**	**738**	**3,799**	**3,096**	**2,249**	**7,836**	**2,723**	**1,146**	**2,315**	**864**	**26,559**

Data collated from returns submitted by district level facilities.

Key to regions: WR= Western, CR= Central, GAR= Greater Accra, VR= Volta, ER= Eastern, ASH=Ashanti,

BAR= Brong Ahafo, NR= Northern, UER= Upper East, UWR= Upper West

Data on psychiatric morbidity in outpatient consultations at district health facilities were collated at the regional level under four psychiatric categories: epilepsy, acute psychosis, neurosis, and substance abuse (Table 4.4). However, these data were likely to be a significant underestimate of the true incidence since many districts lacked psychiatric professionals and did not collate data on psychiatric disorders. Differences between regions were therefore more likely to be due to differences in recording of cases, than to true differences in morbidity.

Between 21-50 percent of primary health care clinics were estimated to refer patients presenting with mental disorders to a higher level of care, such as the psychiatric units of the regional hospitals, or the psychiatric hospitals in Accra or Cape Coast. Communication and collaboration between primary health care workers and psychiatric services was poor and the physical health needs of the mentally ill were often neglected. Between 1-20 percent of workers in the district hospitals and primary health care clinics were estimated to have had contact with a traditional or faith healer. However, no records of such contacts were maintained. Collaboration with traditional or faith healers tended to be informal and was largely undocumented.

Training in mental health care for primary care staff

Approximately 7 percent of the training time for medical doctors was devoted to mental health. General nurses undertook a six-week affiliation at the psychiatric hospitals as part of their training. Post-basic medical assistants received only one week's training in mental health. Some training of primary health care workers in mental health had been facilitated by BasicNeeds and an outreach team from Ankaful Psychiatric Hospital.

In terms of refresher training, there were no data available on how many primary health care doctors and non-doctor/non-nurse primary health care workers had received refresher training in mental health in the index year of 2005. However, responses from the qualitative data indicated that in-service training in psychiatry was limited. Many of the primary health care workers interviewed stated that they had

had no training in psychiatry since they completed their initial clinical training.

Psychotropic medication

All mental hospitals, psychiatric units in general hospitals, and outpatient mental health facilities had at least one psychotropic medicine of each therapeutic class (antipsychotic, antidepressant, mood stabilizer, anxiolytic, and anti-epileptic medicines) available in the facility in 2005. However, the range of psychotropic medication available within GHS was limited largely to older generic drugs. The new generation of antipsychotics and antidepressants, as well as mood-stabilising drugs such as Lithium and Sodium Valproate, were not widely available, despite the inclusion of Sodium Valproate and Risperidone in the Essential Medicines List (GHS Essential Medicines List., 2004). There was limited availability of depot antipsychotic medication, especially outside the psychiatric hospitals.

In the qualitative interviews, several respondents indicated that the supply of psychotropic drugs to inpatient and community facilities was often insufficient, leading to shortages of essential medication. When medication was unavailable at the hospital pharmacies and clinics, patients had to purchase the necessary medication at their own expense.

Human rights protection

There was no national body to oversee regular inspections in mental health facilities, to review involuntary admission and discharge procedures, to review complaints, investigation processes and to impose sanctions (e.g. withdraw accreditation, impose penalties, or close facilities that persistently violated human rights). As a result, none of the mental hospitals nor the inpatient psychiatric units and community residential facilities had any review or inspection of the human rights protection of patients in 2005. However, in the following two years of 2006 and 2007, there were inspections of the psychiatric hospitals by the Commission for Human Rights and Administrative Justice, and in 2008 the Parliamentary Sub-Committee on Health also inspected two of the three state psychiatric hospitals. There was no training in the protection of the human rights of patients in the inpatient psychiatric units and community residential facilities in 2005.

Human resources in mental health care

In 2005, the human resources breakdown for mental health care were as follows: 15 psychiatrists, 468 psychiatric nurses, 132 community psychiatric nurses (CPNs) based in the 10 regions covering 69 of the 138 districts, 7 psychologists, 10 medical assistants, 6 social workers, and 1 occupational therapist. Nine of the psychiatrists working for the GHS were officially retired. The distribution of psychiatric nurses per 100,000 people was 6.29 times greater in Accra than in the entire country. The low numbers of psychologists and occupational therapists was largely attributable to the fact that the GHS did not hire psychologists and had no training programmes for occupational therapists. By 2011/2012 there were 18 psychistrists,19 psychologists, 1068 registered mental health nurses (RMNs) and 72 community mental health officers. This added up to 1177 staff trained in mental health. Another 710 worked in mental health although not specially trained in mental health and included doctors, medical assistants, auxilliaries,social workers etc (MOH 2012).

In 2013, the GHS hired 13 more clinical psychologists and posted them to the regions.

Training professionals in mental health

Since approximately 2011, the Kintampo Project has graduated 15 Medical Assistants in Psychiatry, a middle-level resource trained to give care in psychiatry at the district level. In 2012, the GHS accepted approximately 250 psychology graduates in the National Service corps as health educators in mental health to work alongside CPNs at the community level.

Public education and awareness campaigns on mental health

Mental health professionals and NGOs have conducted a few public education and awareness campaigns in mental health in the last five years, such as World Mental Health Day and the 100th anniversary of the Accra Psychiatric Hospital in 2006. The NGO Mind Freedom has held annual 'Mad Pride' marches in Accra since 2006 to raise awareness of mental health and promote the rights of mental health service users. Several respondents reported conducting occasional educational talks on mental health in schools and churches, as well as local radio broadcasts. Others reported providing training in mental health for traditional healers and pastors. Participants reported that campaigns often target adolescents who are at risk of drug abuse. In addition, campaigns are targeted at women of maternal age who are at risk of depression and other disorders related to pregnancy.

There was some coverage of mental health topics in the national newspapers in Ghana. Between1992 and 2005, the most popular national newspaper, the *Daily Graphic,* published 191 articles on mental health. The most commonly reported topics were suicides, drug abuse, charitable donations to psychiatric hospitals and overcrowding, understaffing and poor conditions in the state psychiatric hospitals. In 2004-2006, Doku et al. reported more coverage of the human rights of the mentally ill, including a review of mental health legislation, and calls for an improvement in psychiatric services (Doku, Ae-Ngbise, Akpalu, et al., 2006). Newspaper articles are only accessible to those who read English.

Inter-sectoral collaboration

There was some formal collaboration between the Mental Health Unit and the departments and agencies responsible for primary health care/community health, reproductive health, child and adolescent health, substance abuse, education, criminal justice and social welfare. However, there was no collaboration with programmes for HIV/AIDS, child protection, employment, housing and the elderly.

In terms of support for child and adolescent health, no primary and secondary schools had either a part-time or full-time mental health professional. However, it was estimated that between 1-20 percent of primary and secondary schools had school-based activities to promote mental health and prevent mental disorders in the form of talks and lay counselling.

Mental Health and Poverty

Mental health is absent in the development discourse on poverty in Ghana. For instance, several initiatives for the alleviation of poverty do not expressly target people living with mental illness even though they may be classified as among the most vulnerable and excluded in society. A National Social Protection Strategy was introduced in 2008 to provide social assistance to the 'poor, vulnerable and excluded'. Although it aims to assist the 'extremely poor' and 'severely disabled', it has not yet specifically targeted the mentally ill as needing assistance (Akomea, 2008). This is partly because the mentally ill fell under the Ministry of Health while the policy was implemented by the Ministry of Manpower, Youth and Employment which had oversight over the Department of Social Welfare.

There are very limited social welfare benefits available in Ghana, two of which were introduced between 2006 and 2008. The District Poverty Alleviation Fund was available for those facing severe economic hardship. Social welfare departments could also make discretionary payments to the destitute, for example meeting their emergency medical costs. Since the passage of the Disability Act in 2006, the District Assemblies are supposed to dedicate up to 2 percent of their Common Fund (funds dispersed to local government for development projects) to those with disabilities. In 2008, the government introduced the Livelihood Empowerment Against Poverty (LEAP) programme alongside the Social Protection Strategy to provide direct cash transfers to the extremely poor, with additional amounts for households with a 'severely disabled person' (Akomea, 2008). However, whilst people with mental illness are included within the definition of those living with a disability under the Disability Act, mental illness is not readily recognised by many policy makers and implementers as a cause of disability and in the criteria for inclusion in the LEAP programme, the emphasis is on physical disability.

Mental health legislation

The legislation in force regarding mental health in Ghana in 2005 was the Mental Health Decree of 1972 (NRCD 1972). The 1972 decree had provisions for procedures for involuntary admission, including rights to appeal, accreditation of professionals and facilities, enforcement of judicial issues for people with mental illness, and mechanisms to implement the provisions of mental health legislation.

The review of the 1972 legislation utilising the WHO Checklist on Mental Health Legislation identified several areas which were not adequately addressed in the Mental Health Decree. These included inadequate attention to the following human rights provisions for service users: the right to humane treatment; confidentiality and privacy; informed consent; the rights of carers and families of users; competency; capacity and guardianship issues; involuntary admission; and issues of seclusion and restraint. There was little protection of vulnerable groups, including minors and women. There was no provision for financing of mental health care and inadequate promotion of mental health within primary or community-based care. There was insufficient promotion of access to psychotropic drugs, and no provision for educational activities, vocational training, leisure activities, and the religious and cultural needs of people with mental disorders. There was no provision made for the involvement of users of mental health services, families and carers in mental health policy and legislation development and planning.

The new Mental Health Law, Act 846, was first drafted in 2006 with support from the WHO (GOG Mental Health Bill 2006). It was enacted in June 2012. Act 846 adopts a human rights approach to mental health, in accordance with the United Nations Charter on Human Rights and international consensus on the health care needs of a person with mental disorder. The law aims to prevent discrimination and provide equal opportunities for people with mental disorder. It addresses many of the weaknesses of the Decree, providing for a mental health authority, a mental health review tribunal, and the protection of the rights of people with mental disorder, including the principle of the least restrictive environment and the right to information and participation. The law, even it its draft form was endorsed by WHO as reflecting best practice in mental health legislation (WHO, 2007). It promotes decentralisation and community mental health care and regulates traditional and faith-based healing practices. An element missing in the law, and identified by the WHO checklist is, that although there is mention of the sources of funding for the mental health authority, there is no stipulation on minimum funding requirements for mental health care or the source of funding. Funding sources, in effect, remain unfinished business for the parliamentary sub-committee on Finance. The implementation of Act 846 has remained a challenge. The Mental Health Board was set up 18 months after the passage of the law without specified funding for the Mental Health Authority

Discussion

The results of the 2005 situation analysis revealed that mental health care in Ghana was comparable with that of many other low-income countries in Africa which show similar patterns of inadequate resources expended largely on institutional care (Jacob et al., 2007; Desjarlais, Eisenberg, Good, et al., 1995). The research reveals continued reliance on the inpatient and outpatient services of the national psychiatric hospitals, despite a policy of decentralisation and a commitment in principle to community mental health care.

Mental health care in Ghana falls far short of WHO's suggested principles for the organization of services, namely accessibility, comprehensiveness, coordination and continuity of care, effectiveness, equity, and respect for human rights (WHO, 2003). WHO suggests that the optimal mix of mental health services may be conceptualized as a pyramid with most, at the base of the pyramid, able to give self-care, while a small minority at the top of the pyramid need to use specialised psychiatric services (WHO, 2003) (see Figure 4.2).

Fig.4.2 **Optimal mix of mental health services (WHO, 2003)**

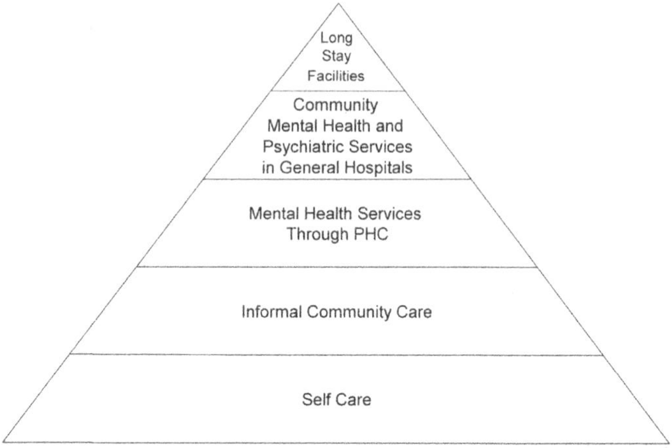

This model proposes that greater numbers of people with mental illness should be treated through informal community care and primary health care, than within specialised community mental health and psychiatric services. Such a model aims to ensure that specialised resources are targeted to those most in need, and that everyone who needs treatment for mental disorders has access to the appropriate level of care. Given the limited resources for mental health in Ghana, and the inequitable spread of services, we consider how the different levels of this pyramid could be implemented in Ghana, maximising the resources available at each level.

Self Care

The situation analysis showed that there is a lack of awareness of mental health and illness among many in Ghana and few public education programmes for mental health. There is, therefore, a need to empower people to give self-care through an active public mental health education programme. Topics should include causes, symptoms, and prevention of mental illness, access to treatment and government programmes on disability and poverty alleviation, and safeguarding patient rights.

Support for families through education and carers' groups would assist families in caring for family members with mental illness. Such programmes have proved successful in India and China (Murthy, Kumar, Chisholm, et al., 2005; Ran, Xiang, Chan, et al., 2003) and carers' groups have been initiated by BasicNeeds and Mind Freedom in Ghana, but there is a need to scale up such interventions nationally.

Informal Community Care

Informal community care in Ghana is offered through faith and traditional healers. Human rights abuses by these healers have been reported, however they remain very popular. Many Ghanaians approach faith and traditional healers for both common mental disorders such as anxiety and moderate mood disorders (Osei, 2001) as well as the more severe psychoses (Read, 2012).

There have been few attempts to develop and supervise the services of traditional and faith healers in Ghana (Montia, 2008; Ventevogel, 1996). In order to reduce the abuse of people with mental illness within informal treatment facilities, a mental health authority and tribunal must be established as stipulated in the new Mental Health Law to regulate the practices of traditional and faith healers. Closer collaboration between faith and traditional healers and orthodox psychiatric care could help to protect the human rights of those with mental illness and ensure that those who would benefit from psychiatric treatment are referred to appropriate services. Initiatives by BasicNeeds to work with traditional healers in northern Ghana have suggested the potential for successful collaboration (Montia, 2008). There is a need to provide training for traditional and faith healers on mental health, psychiatric treatment, ethics and human rights. Local government at the district level (District Assemblies) could help by providing some funding to upgrade the facilities of faith and traditional healers to further improve care given to patients (Ofori-Atta, Akpalu, Osei & Doku, 2007).

In addition, there is a large number of Community-Based Surveillance Volunteers (CBSVs) and Traditional Birth Attendants (TBAs) who are posted to mainly rural communities. WHO calls them 'local experts' (WH0, 2003), who as frontline workers can direct community members to appropriate healthcare. The training of such volunteers in mental health could enable them to extend their support services and make appropriate referrals of people with mental illness. There, is however, a need to consider issues of remuneration for such volunteers in order to ensure that they are motivated and committed to carrying out their work effectively.

Mental Health Services through Primary Health Care

The integration of mental health into primary health care services would ensure that those with mild and moderate mental disorders are able to access care through primary health care facilities, with referral to specialist services only for those with severe symptoms. This would require training primary health care workers in the detection and treatment of mental disorders, and providing regular supervision by mental health professionals. There should be reliable access to psychotropic medication at the district and sub-district level and effective systems of referral and back-referral between primary care and specialised mental health services. Mental health should also be included within the wider public health care initiatives of district health services such as maternal, child, and adolescent health.

There is a need to strengthen the mental health information system in primary care to enable more efficient planning and resource allocation for mental health. In addition, multi-sectoral district mental health advisory committees should be established to apromote mental health within relevant sectors such as education, the police and judiciary, social services, and faith and traditional healers.

Community Mental Health and Psychiatric Services in General Hospitals

As the results show, only 69 of the 138 districts had community psychiatric nurses. Even where a CPN service was provided, there were often only one or two nurses for the district, and they had no access to transportation. Therefore, the service was severely limited in its ability to reach those in need. For years, the number of CPNs in active service diminished as many were near retirement and there was no programme for their replacement. The CPN training programme has been restarted by the MOH while a new middle-level cadre of community mental health workers (see http://thekintampoproject.squarespace.com) will enable the expansion of community mental health care. Strengthening the provision of community mental health services, ensuring an adequate and reliable supply of psychotropic drugs, as well as the provision of transport for community health workers, would improve access to treatment within the community and help prevent the need for hospital admission for many. The hiring of allied mental health professionals, such as psychologists, for districts in 2013 marks a real change for the better.

Access to treatment at the community level is particularly important in Ghana since many communities are far from inpatient psychiatric services which are located in only half of the regional capitals. Many patients bypass these and are admitted to the large psychiatric hospitals in the south, meaning treatment is even further from the person's home. This has implications for the reintegration of the person into his or her community following discharge, particularly given the frequently lengthy admissions and the stigma associated with the psychiatric hospitals. A model of collaboration between one district health service and a prayer camp is currently being studied by the University of Ghana Medical School and Yale University to see how best to utilize this unique community resource while reducing the incidence of human rights abuses.

Psychiatric units should be opened in general hospitals in the remaining regions, and systems of referral and back-referral with primary care strengthened so that use of the regional units is maximised. More beds should be provided at the regional psychiatric units in order to aid the process of de-institutionalisation of the psychiatric hospitals and provision of care nearer home.

In 2012 and 2013, graduates with training in clinical and community psychology from the University of Ghana were posted to do national service with community psychriatric nurses in a pilot called the Psycho Corps Project (Ofori-Attah, Bradley & Nyonaor, 2013). They were primarily to engage in mental health care education in communities and support families with mental illness. If this pilo project is successful, it will mean more young people will be engaged in mental health services and could lead to reduction of stigma towards the mentally ill.

Specialist Services

De-institutionalisation was required to reduce the numbers of long-stay patients in the psychiatric hospitals so as to offer more humane, high-quality care for those most in need. From 2010, Accra and Pantang Psychiatric hospitals reduced their patient numbers by approximately a third to a half. This has been achieved through deliberate actions on the part of the hospitals' CPNs and social workers to re-unite patients with their family as well as the recent creation of brief assessment units in each of these two hospitals which provide for patients to be assessed over three nights before admission is granted if necessary. Otherwise patients are treated, given medication and linked with CPN services close to their homes.

There is also a need for greater diversity within specialized services. At present, inpatient care is largely medicinal with little attention to psychosocial interventions. Halfway houses and vocational rehabilitation could help with the process of de-institutionalisation, particularly for those long-stay patients who are estranged from their families and are in need of a graded reintroduction to life within the community.

It is also time to set up child and adolescent mental health services and particularly urgently needed services are rehabilitation centres for the addictive disoders.

Information systems

The completion of the WHO-AIMS, which relies on data collection by government, private and voluntary services, revealed some of the weaknesses of the health information system particularly, with respect to mental health, in which much data is not gathered at all, or is inconsistent or unreliable. This highlights the need for the introduction of a standardised and comprehensive mental health information system in order to provide the necessary evidence for scaling-up mental health services in Ghana. Crucial to the success of the new Mental Health Law is the collection of accurate routine data which will inform relevant institutions about the use of services and the protection of the rights of users. From a legal point of view, therefore, strengthening of the mental health information system is an urgent necessity (see the last section of this book for a description of the Mental Health Information System and a pilot to improve the system in the three psychiatric hospitals).

Funding

In low-income countries, cost-effective health care is a major priority. A number of studies on the cost-effectiveness of community care for mental disorders in low-income countries have been published (Wiley-Exley, 2004; Gureje, Chisholm, Kola et al., 2007; Chisholm, Lund, Saxena, 2007; Pate, Chisholm, Rabe-Hesketh et al., 2003). It has been calculated that scaling-up mental healthcare in low-income countries would cost around $2-3 per person per year (Chisholm et al., 2007). This is based on a core package for the treatment of schizophrenia, bipolar affective disorder, depression and hazardous alcohol use in which the majority of people with these conditions are treated within district level mental health services and primary care.

One area of the new law which needs more thought is how to fund improvements in mental health services so as not to leave funding to the discretion of budget officers, and ministers of health and finance. Given the low priority of mental health, this raises the risk that mental health may be overlooked. In principle, the process of de-institutionalisation ought to release some funding for community mental health care, and this should be ring-fenced for investment in mental health care. However, as WHO points out, there may be a need for added significant investment in such aspects as training, personnel, and transport, particularly at the onset, to establish mental health within primary care (WHO 2003).

Conclusion

This chapter provides a comprehensive review of mental health policy and service provision in Ghana, and charts a way forward for the development of mental health care. Crucial to this is the implementation of the new law which promises to be a significant step forward in the transformation of mental health care in Ghana.

Acknowledgements
We would like to acknowledge the support of the Ghana Health Service, particularly Dr. Akwasi Osei, in conducting this study. We gratefully acknowledge the assistance of Dr.Victor Doku, Mr. Bright Akpalu, Mr. Kenneth Ae-Ngebise and Mr. Daniel Awenva in the data collection and analysis. This research was funded by the Department for International Development (DfID). The views expressed are not necessarily those of DfID. We thank Hon. Frema Opare, former Deputy Minister of Manpower Youth and Employment for her helpful comments on disability and the LEAP, and Dr. Ahmed, retired Director of Medical Services, for his comments on funding and the Mental Health Bill.

References

Asare, J.B. (2003). Mental Health Profile, Ghana. Place: Publisher.

Bolton, P., Bass, J., Neugebauer, R. et al. (2003). Group Interpersonal Psychotherapy for Depression in Rural Uganda: A Randomized Controlled Trial. *Journal of the American Medical Association*;289 (23):3117-3124.

Chisholm, D., Lund, C., Saxena S. (2007). Cost of scaling up mental healthcare in low- and middle-income countries. *The British Journal of Psychiatry*;**191**(6):528-535.

Desjarlais, R., Eisenberg, L., Good. B., and Kleinman A. (1995) *World Mental Health: Problems and Priorities in Low-Income Countries*. Oxford University Press.

Diop, D. & Dores, M. (1976) L'admission d'un acccompagnant du malade à l'hôpital psychiatrique. *African Journal of Psychiatry*;**1**:119-130.

Doku, V.C.K., Ae-Ngbise, K., Akpalu, B, Read, U.M. and Anum, A. (2006) Portrayal of mental illness in a Ghanaian national newspaper: A prospective study. Paper presented at the 3rd International Mental Health Conference. London, UK.

Flisher, A.J., Lund, C., Funk, M., Banda, M., Bhana, A., Doku, V., Drew, N., Kigozi, F.N., Knapp, M., Omar, M., Petersen, I. and Green, A. (2007). Mental health policy development and implementation in four African countries. *J Health Psychol.* 12(3):505-516.PMID:17440000[

Franklin, R.R., Sarr, D., Gueye, M., Sylla, O., Collignon, R. (1996). Cultural response to mental illness in Senegal: Reflection through patient companions - Part 1. Methods and descriptive data. *Social Science and Medicine*;42(3):325-338.

Ghana Health Service. 2004. *Standard Treatment Guidelines.*

Ghana Health Service. 2004.*Essential Medicines List.*

Ghana Statistical Service (2003). Ghana Demographic and Health Survey. Ghana Statistical Service and Noguchi Memorial Institute for Medical Research, Legon, Accra,.

Government of Ghana (2007). The Implementation of the Growth and Poverty Reduction Strategy (GPRS II): 2006 Annual Progress Report. Accra,

Government of Ghana.(2006). Disability Act.

Gureje, O., Chisholm, D., Kola, L., Lasebikan, V., Saxena, S. (2007). Cost effectiveness of an essential mental health intervention package in Nigeria. *World Psychiatry*;6:42-48.

Jacob, K.S., Sharan, P., Mirza, I., Garrido-Cumbrera, M., Seedat, S., Mari, J.J., Sreenivas, V., Saxena, S. (2007). Mental health systems in countries: where are we now? *The Lancet* 370:1061-1077.

Kilonzo, G.P. and Simmons N. Development of mental health services in Tanzania: A reappraisal for the future(1998). *Social Science and Medicine*;47(4):419-428.

Kohn, R., Saxena ,S., Levav, I., Saraceno, B. (2004). The treatment gap in mental health care. *Bulletin of the World Health Organization;*82:858-866.

Montia, S. Fostering productive partnerships with traditional healers. Mental Health and Development (2008). http://www.mentalhealthanddevelopment.org/files/Traditional%20Healers%20Article.pdf Accessed on 9th October 2008.

Murthy, R.S., Kumar, K.V.K., Chisholm, D., Thomas,T., Sekar, K., Chandrashekar, C.R. (2005). Community outreach for untreated schizophrenia in rural India: a follow-up study of symptoms, disability, family burden and costs. *Psychological Medicine*;35:341-351.

National Redemption Council Ghana. Mental Health Decree, 1972.

Ofori-Atta A, Akpalu B, Osei AO, Doku VCK (2007). What happens when your mental health fails and society wants you out? A critical study of available options in mental health services around Ghana. Paper presented at the Scientific Conference of the College of Health Sciences, University of Ghana. Accra, Ghana.

Ofori-Attah A., Bradley, E., Nyonator, F., (2013) Increasing Access to Primary Mental Health Care through task shifting; embracing a new cadre of graduates in psychology in primary health care in Ghana. Paper presentation, Scientific Conference, Centre for Global Mental Health, Institute of Psychiatry, London.

Osei, A.O. (2001)Types of psychiatric illness at traditional healing centres in Ghana. *Ghana Medical Journal*; 35(3):106-110.

Patel, V., Chisholm, D., Rabe-Hesketh, S., Dias-Saxena, F., Andrew, G., Mann, A. (2003). Efficacy and cost-effectiveness of drug and psychological treatments for common mental disorders in general health care in Goa, India: a randomised, controlled trial. *The Lancet* 361:33-39.

Patel, V. Poverty, inequality, and mental health in developing countries. In: Leon, D.A, Walt, G., (Eds.). (2001):. *Poverty, Inequality and Health: An International Perspective.* Oxford: Oxford University Press, 247-262.

Patel, V., Araya, R., Chatterjee, S., Chisholm, D., Cohen, A., De Silva, M., Hosman, C., McGuire, H., Rojas, G., van Ommeren, M. (2007). Treatment and prevention of mental disorders in low-income and middle-income countries. *The Lancet*;370:44-58.

Patel, V. and Kleinman, A. (2003). Poverty and common mental disorders in developing countries. *Bulletin of the World Health Organization*;81(8):609-615.

Ran, M-S., Xiang, M-Z., Chan, CL-W., Leff, J., Simpson, P., · Huang, M-S., Shan, Y-H., Li, S-G. (2003). Effectiveness of psychoeducational intervention for rural Chinese families experiencing schizophrenia. *Social Psychiatry and Psychiatric Epidemiology*; 38(2):69-75.

Read, U.M.(2012) Chains and Vagrancy; Living with Mental Illness in Kin tampo, Ghana. Unpublished PHD thesis, University College, London.

Ritchie, J., Spencer, L. (1994). Qualitative data analysis for applied policy research. In: Bryman A, Burgess RG, eds. Analysing Qualitative Data. Routledge, London: 173-194.

Saraceno, B., Levav, I., & Kohn, R. (2005;). The public mental health significance of research on socio-economic factors in schizophrenia and major depression. *World Psychiatry* 4(3):181-185.

Saxena, S., Thornicroft, G., Knapp, M., Whiteford, H. (2007). Resources for mental health: scarcity, inequity and inefficiency. *The Lancet*;370:878-889.

Sefa-Dedeh, A., Ofori-Atta, A., Ohene, S., Baah-Odoom, D. (2006). A model of integration of research with mental health care provision in the Upper West Region: An observational study of patient-staff interaction in two hospitals in the Upper-West Region. The Annual Conference of the College of Health Sciences, University of Ghana. Accra, Ghana.

Siskind, D., Bolton, P., and Kim, J. (2007). Country contextualization of cost-effectiveness: Analysis of treatments for depression in Chile and Uganda using a Markov model. *Journal of Mental Health Policy and Economics* ;10:S40-S41.

Twumasi, P.A. (1979). Community Involvement in Health Care: The Kintampo Experience in Ghana. A Study in the Changing Health Model. *Ghana Medical Journal*:80-84.

United Nations Development Programme. (2005). Human Development Index.

Ventevogel, P. (1996) *Whiteman's Things: Training and De-training Healers in Ghana*. Amsterdam: Het Spinhuis,

WHO (2001). *The World Health Report: Mental Health: New Understanding, New Hope*. Geneva: World Health Organization.

WHO (2002). Nations for Mental Health: Final Report. Geneva: World Health Organization.

WHO (2005). WHO Assessment Instrument for Mental Health Systems (WHO-AIMS) Version 2.2. World Health Organization, Geneva,.

WHO (2005.)Resource Book on Mental Health, Human Rights and Legislation. World Health Organization, Geneva.

WHO (2003). Organization of Services for Mental Health. Mental Health Policy and Services Guidance Package. Geneva: World Health Organization.

WHO.(2007) Ghana Country Summary. Mental Health Improvement for Nations Development (MIND). Geneva: World Health Organization..

WHO (2005) WHO Resource Book on Mental Health, Human Rights and Legislation. World Health Organization, Geneva,

Wiley-Exley E. (2007) Evaluations of community mental health care in low- and middle-income countries: A 10-year review of the literature. *Social Science & Medicine*; 64 (6):1231-1241.

Endnote

1. First published in the African Journal of Psychiatry in 2010, (13, 99-108) Reprinted here with permission from the Publishers, with updates on Act 846, Mental Health Law 2012.

Section B

Conceptualization of Mental Illness

Chapter 5

The Ghanaian Non-Medical Conceptualization of Mood Disorders

Sammy Ohene and Selassie Addom

Depressive disorders constitute a great proportion of mental disorders that affect human beings worldwide. Unipolar and bipolar depression are responsible for a significant amount of morbidity and distress. Sadness as a state of feeling or mood has always been recognized as part of human emotions. Prolonged grief from loss or adversity, akin to descriptions of the depressive state can be found in ancient texts such as the book of Job in the Holy Bible. Whilst depression as a disease entity gained recognition in psychiatric literature, early Western psychiatrists doubted the occurrence of depression among Africans. Carothers (1947) categorically stated that depression did not exist among Africans. This view was seriously challenged by Fields (1955) who suggested that most of the women she studied in the then Gold Coast (now Ghana), who confessed to witchcraft, were exhibiting the self-accusatory symptoms often seen in depressed British women. Her belief was confirmed by Osei (2001) who found all 17 women in three shrines who had confessed to witchcraft, suffered from depression according to ICD-10 criteria. Fields, in fact, declared depression to be the commonest mental disorder among rural *Akan* women (Fields, 1960).

Majodina and Johnson (1983) demonstrated that depression could be diagnosed among Ghanaians utilizing the same instruments as in Western cultures. Using the Schedule of Affective and Depressive Disorders (SADD), they found in a small study of 50 patients, 40 reported somatic symptoms like headaches, body heat and general bodily pains. Many respondents in the study also reported anxiety, tension, guilt, loss of interest, inability to enjoy themselves and sadness. In another study, Turkson and Dua (1997) utilized the Montgomery-Asberg Depressive Rating Scale (M-ADRS) with 131 depressed female patients at the Accra Psychiatric Hospital. They found a high level of somatic complaints like headaches (77.9 percent) and sleeplessness (68.7 percent), but relatively low incidence of psychological symptoms like sadness(13 percent) and pessimistic thoughts (20.6 percent), with 7.3 percent of the depressed women admitting to suicidal ideas.

Perez and Junot (1998) stated that depression in Africans presented in a mode specific to African culture involving the individual and his relationship to others. In their view, the Western model of depression was irrelevant to Africa, but predicted that with increasing modernization, features of the disorder would tend to look more like, and have outcomes similar to those seen in Western countries.

Depression is characterized by the presence of symptoms like sadness, loss of interest, loss of self-confidence, inappropriate guilt feelings as well as thoughts of death and suicide. Invariably, depressed individuals have disturbances of sleep, appetite and impaired concentration. Additionally in many populations including among Ghanaians, depressed individuals present with multiple bodily complaints. In fact, the somatic symptoms may be so overwhelming they may appear to obscure the core depressive symptoms. Whilst many of these symptoms may sometimes occur after adverse life events, a diagnosis of clinical depression is made only after persistence of the symptoms over a minimum of two weeks. (American Psychiatric Association, 2006; World Health Organization, 1992). Depression may be mild, moderate or severe in intensity and often runs a recurrent course. However, up to 20% of patients have depression that is chronic and non-remitting, (Thornicroft & Sartorious, 1993).

To understand the effects of depression on the human being, it is helpful to think of depression as a disease that affects the brain and disrupts all cerebral functions. Depressed patients often have slowed heart rate and blood pressure leading to dizziness. Digestive secretions reduce causing constipation. Frequent complaints of various types of pain and irritability occur due to reduced pain and noise threshold. Slowed motor activity and muscle fatigue is often seen. Sleep and hormonal functions are disrupted leading to menstrual abnormalities in women for example. Higher cognitive functions such as memory, attention and reasoning capacity are all compromised. (Moussaoui, 2012).

Depression occurs all over the world. Analysis of the ***Global burden of disease*** 2000 study, estimates the point prevalence of depression worldwide to be 1.9 percent in men and 3.2 percent in women. Over a twelve- month period, 5.8 percent of men and 9.5 percent of women would be expected to experience depression. Unipolar depression is the fourth leading cause of burden among all diseases. It is responsible for a huge proportion of working time lost in the age group 15-44, accounting for the second highest burden of disease worldwide, with 8.5 percent of DALYs lost. (WHO, 2006). A recent study in Ghana estimated the cost of this psychological distress to Ghana was equivalent to 7 percent of GDP (Canauvan, Spsma, Adhuaryu, et al, 2013).

Often overlooked is the significantly reduced output by depressed individuals even when they struggle to work, probably because of their markedly impaired concentration.

Like all mental disorders, depression evokes much stigma and puts enormous strain on the families of affected individuals too. These include emotional stress of coping with disturbed behavior, restriction of social activities and the economic burden of treatment costs (WHO, 1997).

A serious and tragic complication of depression is suicide with some studies suggesting as much as 15-20 percent of sufferers may commit suicide. (Goodwin & Jamieson, 1990).

Presentation of depression in Ghanaians

There is no known word in any Ghanaian language that specifically describes the syndrome clinically described as depression. Most affected people focus on the physical or somatic symptoms that are manifest in the disorder. Common among these are complaints of headaches, usually described as of a burning nature or feeling of heat inside the head. The headaches may also be characterized as feeling of heaviness or tension. Frequent complaints are pain in various body parts, often migratory and following no particular anatomical configuration, as well as feelings of crawling movements all over the body. Ghanaians with depressive disorders also tend to emphasize their sleep symptoms like insomnia, 'bad' dreams and nightmares.

It must be stressed, as shown above, that the other core features of depression like loss of interest, poor concentration, lowered self-esteem and guilt feelings do occur in Ghanaians. Very often however, these have to be elicited by the clinician unlike the other symptoms that are usually reported spontaneously. It is not uncommon to hear complaints of "thinking too much" and having "bad thoughts" from depressed persons or a frustrated expression of feeling "***basaa***" after a long struggle to find the right words to explain their mood. The interpretations of these various symptoms appear to give some insights into the Ghanaian's understanding of the disorder classified as depression.

Most complaints of headaches and other bodily pains in depressed people are initially regarded as due to malaria, assumed to be the commonest cause of such symptoms in Ghana. Patients may self-medicate and/or go through several treatment courses with anti-malarial drugs and other medications from clinicians they see before a diagnosis of depression is made. In many cases, various investigations including scans and biochemical tests may have been carried out, yielding no "positive" results.

The lack of improvement in the symptoms of a depressed person after such treatment and the inability to identify specific visible lesions on medical tests reinforces the belief of many such people that their illness has no physical or organic cause. For many Ghanaians, a medical consultation should identify an illness with a clearly known physical cause and a treatment which cures the malady. The inability of modern medicine to meet these expectations (at least before the patient gets expert psychiatric care) leads to a belief that the symptoms have a *spiritual* cause.

Many individuals with depression tend to link their symptoms to *witchcraft, curses,* and similar supernatural causes. This belief is supposed to explain why the character of headaches for example, is unlike the more common throbbing pain associated with malaria. A crawling sensation inside or on the body is often assumed to be due to worm infestation and many of the patients take or demand anti-helminthic medications repeatedly.

Patients who look or sound depressed may admit or deny feeling depressed. Some do not believe in being intrinsically depressed and seek to rationalize their low mood by attributing it to their physical symptoms like headaches or sleeplessness. Many express ideas like "if only I could sleep, all my problems would go". Others do not accept a feeling of depression in the absence of an obvious environmental cause and even crying spells are taken to be due to a physical symptom instead of a low emotional state.

The phrase directly translated from many Ghanaian languages as '*thinking too much*' when explored further turns out to be an expression of *obsessive rumination*. It is a common symptom often missed by most clinicians but is often present in many patients who admit to waking up late at night, unable to resume sleep with their minds filled with unwanted thoughts. Closely linked to this is the complaint of '*bad thoughts*'. This indicates the presence of negative thoughts usually of a morbid nature or thoughts considered blasphemous or sacrilegious. Ghanaians are known to be extremely religious. The 2010 census reported over 94.3% of people claimed adherence to one or other religion such as Christianity, Islam or traditional worship, (Ghana Statistical Service, 2012). Patients are particularly reluctant to verbalize thoughts of suicide even when these thoughts assume an obsessive character, preferring the euphemism *bad thoughts*. By their religious persuasion a lot of Ghanaians believe that suicide will lead to eternal damnation in the afterlife and so would normally not consider the act even when the idea persistently intrudes into their minds. Suicidal ideation, as well as all the peculiar complaints mentioned earlier must therefore be carefully elicited in all depressed patients since they will very rarely report it spontaneously.

The following case reports of patients illustrate the peculiar presentation of depression in Ghana.

Case 1: Mr. AT.

64 year-old Mr. AT, a pharmacist, presented with a history of a feeling of worms moving in his body for one and half years. He had taken several doses of albendazole and ivermectin (anti-parasitic agents) but had seen little improvement. Some months later, he said, some

demons started attacking the worms but also attacked some of his internal organs as well till his heart and stomach had been completely eaten away. He believed a foreign object had been implanted in his body to function as his heart and when he ate the food went straight to his feet. He also had insomnia, anorexia, feelings of hopelessness and worthlessness as well as social withdrawal. Prior to referral, he had done several investigations which were all normal. He had no past history of mental illness and no chronic illness.

His father was dead but his mother alive with dementia. He had lost his wife 9 years prior to presentation. He had 3 children, 2 of whom lived with him at home but were not supportive. His older brother, who lived close to him, took care of his meals and accompanied him for his hospital visits. He had been working throughout the course of the illness.

Physical examination was normal. Mental state examination revealed a well dressed man sitting calmly. His mood was depressed but affect appropriate. Speech was slow with a low tone, though relevant. He had paranoid and nihilistic delusions but no hallucinations. His orientation was good, and attention sustained but concentration was impaired. Memory was normal.

A diagnosis of depression with psychotic symptoms was made and he was treated accordingly.

His symptoms improved significantly on follow-up visits.

Case 2: Mr CC

26 year-old Mr. CC, an immigrant from one of the neighboring countries, had been living in Ghana for 5 years. He presented with the sensation of "something" crawling all over his body which started soon after his move to Ghana and a 2 year history of biting sensation all over his body. He had visited several hospitals and done several investigations including HIV tests which were all normal. He had difficulty falling asleep, anorexia and weight loss but no suicidal thoughts or anhedonia.

He had been started on treatment for depression about 9 months prior to presentation but he only took the medication for a month and stopped because he did not feel an improvement in his symptoms.

There was no significant past medical history.

CC was single and had no children. The 2nd of 6 children, both his parents were alive and well. He was a trader in car spare parts and lived with 2 of his brothers. He drank alcohol occasionally and had smoked cannabis for about 4 months, 5 years earlier.

Physical examination was essentially normal. Mental state examination revealed a neat and calm looking young man. He had a depressed mood with appropriate affect. His speech, thought stream, form and possession were normal. He expressed the belief that something was biting his insides and sucking his blood. This belief however did not have the intensity of a delusion. Cognition was intact.

A diagnosis of depression was made, with the possibility of somatization disorder considered. Setraline (an antidepressant drug) was prescribed. He however did not return for follow up.

Case 3: Ms AA

35 year-old Ms AA is a finance officer, single mother of one child. She presented with the sensation of something crawling up her vagina for a year and a 2 month history of poor sleep. She frequently experienced this sensation in her vagina when she was at work and the air conditioner was on or when a male colleague entered the room. It sometimes occurred when alone walking along a road. Her appetite had increased; she felt like eating everything in sight. She had become socially withdrawn, felt worthless and had recurrent thoughts of suicide but had made no attempts. She had low energy and difficulty getting out of bed in the mornings.

She had no known chronic illness but had had a breast lump removed about 10 years earlier.

She was the 5th of 6 children, all of whom and their parents were alive and well. There was no reported family history of mental illness.

She had been in a non-consensual relationship arranged by her parents and pastor from which she had an 8 year old son. She had endured multiple incidents of sexual abuse over the past year but had not reported any of them.

She drank alcohol occasionally and did not smoke nor was there a history of psychoactive substance use. Physical examination was normal. Mental state examination revealed a well dressed but timid looking young woman. She was fidgety and unable to maintain eye contact. Mood was depressed and affect appropriate but speech was slow and low toned. Her thought processes were normal and no disorders of perception were noted. She was well oriented in time, person and place and attention was sustained. Concentration was impaired but memory was intact and she had good insight.

A diagnosis of depression was made. She was put on amitriptyline and psychotherapy started.

Patient had improved when reviewed after a month.

Case 4: Ms. MA

22 year-old Ms MA, a shop attendant, presented with a 2 month history of a sensation of worms crawling out of her nostrils, ears and through her vagina. She also felt them crawling all over her body and sometimes felt the worms squeezing her breasts. She had taken different worm expellants but felt no relief. Her brothers were also said to have seen her talking to herself, especially at night, sometimes with gestures. She had insomnia, anorexia and weight loss. She attributed her weight loss to the worms sucking her blood. M.A did not have any feelings of hopelessness or worthlessness but felt very sad 'because of the worms'. She had no suicidal thoughts and was able to attend to her daily activities. She had no previous mental illness and no chronic physical illness.

Her parents were divorced. She was the 3rd of 7 children, comprising 6 half siblings, 3 from each parent, all of whom were alive and well. There was no reported family history of mental illness.

She had lived with her father and stepmother during her childhood, a childhood described as generally good though there were times she felt her father had been hard on her whilst her stepmother sided with him.

Her father stopped paying her school fees when she got pregnant in form 2 of senior high school, whereupon she dropped out of school. She eventually terminated the pregnancy with the help of her boyfriend. At the time of presentation she was not in an intimate relationship and lived with her mother.

Physical examination was essentially normal. Mental state examination revealed a well-dressed young woman, sitting calmly. Her mood was depressed, affect was appropriate with speech of normal volume and rate. Thought processes were normal with the exception of the delusion of being infested by worms. She did not admit to hearing voices but admitted she had been talking in her sleep since childhood. There was no cognitive impairment but she lacked insight.

A diagnosis of depression was made and treatment was started. However she did not return for follow up.

Management of depression

Many people suffering from depression believe their condition is due to a physical ailment. The feelings of depression are considered to be a reaction to the worrying and often long-standing bodily complaints to which they cannot find a cure. The failure to identify specific organic diseases or indeed a causative organism for the symptoms adds to the frustration of the depressed individual. For the Ghanaian, this situation may further strengthen the belief that the symptoms result from supernatural causes, for which reason laboratory investigations and imaging techniques appear to draw blank or "negative" results.

Well thought out and targeted investigations may actually prove therapeutic. A negative result can allay the patient's fears about having a serious disease like cancer.

The proper management of a depressed patient must start with a detailed explanation of the disorder to the affected person. A biopsychosocial model is often useful in relating the interaction between environmental and intrinsic factors to induce changes in body function which in turn may manifest as symptoms. The approach is not always convincing to those with strong culturally held views on the causes of their condition. For such people it is perhaps more helpful to accept their beliefs and work with or around them.

A patient who believes in carrying out a symbolic sacrifice or offering to appease the offended deities or individuals for example, will not be discouraged. Such actions may considerably reduce anxiety and aid recovery efforts. On the contrary, the patient's symptoms may be rationalized as the pathway through which the supernatural forces are acting and whatever will give relief should be helpful.

In general, three broad modalities of treatment are used in the care of patients suffering from depression. These are *psychological, environmental and physical.*

The psychological approach considered most effective is **Cognitive Behavior Therapy (CBT).** This was pioneered by Beck (1979). CBT should be administered by a trained person. The lack of people skilled in its use limits the application of CBT to very few centers in Ghana such as our own department of Psychiatry, UGMS and the Military Hospital with Wuzuame, a trained cognitive behavior therapist and a physician.

Attempting to resolve or directly cope with practical environmental stressors like poverty, abusive relationships and stressful work situations for example may help a depressed person recover. Many times, the depressive condition induces a state of helplessness and inaction, and the professional caregiver has to provide the impetus that leads to change in the environmental condition. In practice many identifiable negative environmental stressors are difficult to remove and a compromise may be required.

Medications called ***antidepressants*** are the most useful in the care of persons suffering from depression. In Ghana they assume particular importance because most people who attend hospitals for any type of condition expect to be given some medication. The challenge is in administering antidepressants which by their nature, have to be taken for many months to show the desired outcome and many of which have uncomfortable side effects. This requires patience on the part of both patient and prescriber. Properly utilized, antidepressant medications are very useful in alleviating symptoms of the majority of those who need them. They are the mainstay of treatment given for depression in psychiatric facilities, community programmes and even general hospitals. Common causes for failure of treatment with antidepressants are wrong (usually under) dosing and too short duration of treatment.

There are other physical treatments such as ECT (electroconvulsive therapy) and TMS (transcranial magnetic stimulation) available in specialized facilities that are used for care of more resistant cases of depression.

Commentaries on case illustrations

Case No. 1

The presenting complaints that emphasize bodily symptoms of a physical nature are now well recognized as being typical of depression in many cultures (Tylee & Ghandi, 2005; Turkson & Dua 1996). Such symptoms are very common among Ghanaian and other African patients.

The other symptoms of depressed mood, feelings of hopelessness and worthlessness, anhedonia, social withdrawal, reduced concentration and slowed speech and activity, ongoing for over 2 weeks, more than satisfies diagnostic criteria for depression in the standard diagnostic manuals such as ICD-10 (WHO 1992) and DSM-IV-Text Revision (American Psychiatric Association, 2006). The apparently bizarre belief that his entrails had disappeared is a rare but well documented nihilistic delusion seen in some cases of severe depression also known as *Cotard's syndrome*(Debruyne, Van den Eynde & Audenaert, 2009). The delusions may lead to a misdiagnosis of schizophrenia but the good response to antidepressants and age of the patient make that unlikely for a first episode.

Case No 2.

CC had multiple somatic (bodily) symptoms of crawling and biting sensations. He also had anorexia, weight loss and sleep disturbance. His mood was depressed whilst he believed his blood and internal organs were being consumed. Whilst no other symptoms of major depression were elicited, 3 of the major diagnostic criteria out of a prescribed minimum of 4 are present. These, in addition to somatic symptoms and possibly impaired concentration, not reported but very likely, make a diagnosis of depression very likely. The unrewarding but repeated laboratory investigations illustrate the point about the frequent conviction of many that their symptoms have a physical cause.

Case No 3.

The symptoms diagnostic of depression in this patient are clear and beyond doubt. The sexual connotations of her somatic symptoms are not surprising in view of her experience of sexual abuse in a relationship contracted by coercion that had resulted in the birth of a son.

Case No 4.

This is a case in which the basic requirements for diagnosis of depression are met. There are however, other symptoms suggestive of delusions and possibly hallucinations to which she may be responding to by "talking to herself". These make it necessary to further explore and consider the possibility of other major psychiatric disorders such as schizophrenia. Unfortunately this patient was lost to follow-up. It illustrates the fact that depression may also occur concurrently with or secondary to other conditions, psychiatric or physical.

References

American Psychiatric Association (2000). *Diagnostic and Statistical Manual of Mental Disorders* .4th ed, Text Revision. Washington DC: APR.

Canavan, M., Advharyu, A., et al. (2013). Psychological distress in Ghana: associations with employment and lost productivity. *Int. J. Mental Health Systems.* Article url http//www.ijmhs.com/content/7/1/9.

Carothers, J. C., (1947). A study of mental derangement in Africans and an attempt to explain its pecuriarities more especially in relation to the African attitude in life. *J. Mental Sc.* 97: 12-48.

Beck, A.T., Rush, A.J., Shaw, B.F., & Emery, G. (1979). *Cognitive therapy of depression.* New York: Guilford Press.

Debruyne H, Portzky M, Van den Eynde F, & Audenaert K (2009) Cotard's syndrome: a review. *Curr Psychiatry Rep.* Jun;11(3):197-202.

Fields, M. (1955).Witchcraft as a primitive interpretation of mental disorder. *Journal of Mental Science*; 101;826-33

Fields, M.(1960). *Search for security: An Ethno Psychiatric study of Rural Ghana,* pp 149. London:Faber & Faber.

Majodina, M.Z. & Johnson, Y.F. (1983). Standardized assessment of depressive disorders in Ghana; *Br. J of Psychiatry*;143:442-6

Osei, A.O. (2001). Witchcraft and depression: a study into the psychopathological features of alleged witches. *Ghana Med. J.*;35(3):111-15.

Perez S. & Junot A.(1998). Depression in Sub-Saharan Africa(article in French). *Med. Trop. Mars)*;58(2):168-72.

Tylee, A. & Gandhi P. (2005). The Importance of Somatic Symptoms in Depression in Primary Care. *Prim Care Companion J Clin Psychiatry;* 7(4): 167–176.

Turkson, N.A. and Dua, A.N. (1996). A study of the social and clinical characteristics of depression among Ghanaian women (1982-1992). *West Afr. J. Med.* 15(2):85-90.

World Health Association (1992). *Int. Classification of Dis.*-10.

Chapter 6

Religion and Psychotherapy

Araba Sefa-Dedeh

Introduction

Every culture has its own healing traditions and practices both for physical illness and psychopathology. There are however, similarities among these practices that cross cultures. Jerome Frank (1974), in his study of psychotherapy across cultures has defined it as "those types of influences characterized by:

1. A trained socially sanctioned healer whose healing powers are accepted by the sufferer and by his social group or an important segment of it.
2. A sufferer who seeks relief from the healer.
3. A circumscribed more or less structured series of contacts between the healer and the sufferer, through which the healer often with the aid of a group tries to produce certain changes in the sufferer's emotional state attitudes and behaviour ..... the healer's influence is primarily exercised by words, acts and rituals in which sufferer, healer and – if there is one – group, participate jointly" (p.2)

It is important that both sufferer and healer have similar beliefs concerning the aetiology of the illness and hope that the process they embark on will relieve the suffering. Part of the work of the healer or therapist is to engender such hope in the client or sufferer. This means that the belief systems under which the therapist/healer and client/sufferer operate are of vital importance to the type of treatments that eventually result in healing.

Belief Systems That Influence Therapy: Euro-America

Euro-American psychotherapy is based on a number of theoretical orientations which can be conceptualised as belief systems. Acocella (2000), in her review of Luhmann's book, "Of Two Minds", indicated that Luhmann approached psychiatry and its training as "a collection of beliefs and practises which young trainees are socialized into". There is the psychodynamic system pioneered by Freud that believes that repressed emotions have to be relieved through strategies that increase insight into one's feelings, attitudes and behaviour. Behaviourism, pioneered by Watson, Pavlov, Thorndike, Skinner, and Wolpe help clients on the basis of the belief that abnormal behaviours can be unlearned and new adaptive behaviours learned.

Cognitive therapists believe and persuade their clients that their thoughts, attitudes and belief systems underlie their abnormal feelings and behaviours. Thus, changing one's thoughts and beliefs help relieve suffering and result in behaviour change.

Humanistic and existential therapists believe that given the right type of nurturing environment, sufferers themselves have the ability to explore their feelings and grow towards a deeper understanding of self and a finding of purpose in life.

Family and other group therapists believe that the individual is influenced greatly by his group setting and thus suffering can only be relieved by influencing the entire group for change.

All of these therapies highlight emotional life with little emphasis on spiritual or religious life. This probably stems from a world view that considers religion and belief in the supernatural as rather primitive and simple. Considering the history of psychopathology in Europe and America and attempts to rid it of demonology, this is understandable though it has led to what can be described as "throwing the baby out with the bath water". In the psychotherapy of the 20th century, it was virtually taboo to address the spiritual in therapy. Any attempts by a client to do so would have probably made him/her seem more pathological. For example, if a client said he was being tormented by spirits, he would probably be seen as psychotic and in need of medication.

The landscape is however changing rapidly. Lothstein (2002) in her review of the book "Handbook of Psychotherapy and Religions", indicated that the editors considered the alienation between religion and mental health as ending and that now it would be strange for a competent therapist not to ask questions about the spirituality of his/

her patients. There are instruments to assess spirituality and religion (Anandarajah & Hight, 2001). Dein (2010) cites Blass (2007) and Lawrence and Duggal (2001) as emphasising the need for teaching spirituality in the psychiatry curriculum. Ferrel's (2013) illustrates this change quite succinctly.

Belief Systems That Influence Healing In Ghana

In contrast to Euro-American systems, in traditional Ghanaian society there is no room for a purely naturalistic notion of illness as is the case in most of Africa (Mbiti, 1975). As Twumasi (1974) explains, there is no clear cut conceptual separation of the natural or physical from the supernatural. It is not surprising that psychopathology is seen as caused predominantly by supernatural forces. This is not to say that physical or emotional causes are not considered important but basically the supernatural is what is conceptualized as most important. Psychopathology therefore is often seen as due to an attack by evil spirits emanating from witchcraft. Sometimes the evil spirits may have been invoked by a curse on the individual or the individual's family for hurt or harm done others. The evil spirits may either just attack or actually possess or dwell within the person. Sometimes the attack may not be from evil spirits but from deities whose rules or taboos may have been infringed by the individual or his family. Thus the attack is seen as punishment for guilt (Assimeng, 1989). Folklore indicates that a person who invokes spirits to obtain power or various favours supernaturally and who becomes afraid or who does not obey the rules governing such an invocation or conjuring can become psychotic or "mad". In essence, the spirits they seek to control turn and control them.

The notion of a human spirit being strong or weak is evident in this conceptualization and will be highlighted in the discussion of the integration between traditional and foreign therapies. Also, according to folklore, if a person is being given witchcraft and his/her soul refuses it then either the conflict or the angry witchcraft/evil spirit could cause a psychosis or abnormal behaviour.

The traditional treatment of psychopathology derives from this perception of the aetiology of psychopathology. Thus rituals of exorcism of spirits, rituals for protection and rituals to pacify deities from spirits are used. The treatment usually follows a diagnosis of the cause of the psychopathology and invocation of more powerful spirits or deities, through divination e.g. the throwing of cowries. Pacification and expiation rituals are usually used when it is felt that the individual is guilty for some reason that can run the gamut of having disrupted normal social relationships, e.g. unfaithfulness in a marital relationship, to breaking a taboo of a deity. Protection, pacification and exorcism rituals are used when attack or possession by spirits is diagnosed. These types of therapies are quite common in other parts of Africa (Dopamu, 1985; Fisher, 1998). Assimeng (1989) in his book "Religion and Social Change in West Africa" believes that the central focus of religious activity in African traditional societies seem to be a warding off of evil spirits or what he terms "homhomfi", the Akan term for evil spirit. Traditionally such therapy was done by religious leaders e.g. shrine priests, pastors etc.

Belief systems in modern Ghanaian society are not necessarily all traditional. The majority of people however have a mixture of traditional and "scientific/naturalistic" beliefs (Ofori-Atta & Linden, 1995). Most people feel that worrying too much or using illegal drugs can cause psychopathology. However, they also believe in spiritual/supernatural attacks and invasion. Those who access psychotherapy in a hospital or clinic are usually of this kind or people who have tried healing in the traditional systems but have not received the help they wanted. Often the symptoms that are described are couched within this belief system, "I am being attacked spiritually". "I do not understand what is happening, I think someone is behind it, attacking me with witchcraft" etc. (Sefa-Dedeh, 2001)

The Way Forward:Integrating The Two Systems

How can the mental health professional be of help in this context when training in the field not only ignores but considers such a world view pathological? The first is to understand the belief system and to be willing to explore the individual's thoughts, emotions and behaviours concerning it. Clinical psychologists/psychiatrists, as healers, have areas of expertise. This expertise makes it possible to explore the physical, emotional and social correlates of behaviour. This is essential within a belief system where only the religious is highlighted. However, it is possible and essential that this expertise be integrated into the original belief systems in order that there is consonance between some aspect of the religious world view and the help being offered.

It is only then that healing can be easily accessed. There is also the possibility of convincing the client to change his/her world view and to adopt the therapist's. Though eventually therapy tends to result in clients' world views changing to become closer to the therapists', beginning therapy with this as its main goal is ineffective and usually results in early drop out.

In the traditional belief systems, a person is born with their personality or "***ɔkra***" in Akan. As was stated earlier, folklore indicates that witches can attack someone with a weak ***ɔkra*** more than a strong one. Certain rituals are also known to strengthen a person spiritually e.g. in Akan the phrase "w'aben ne ho" (Danquah, 1968) is used to signify one steeped in the use of spiritual power.

Therapy that bridges traditional and "scientific" thinking can then be construed as a way of strengthening personality internally rather than externally e.g. with the use of protective devices like amulets etc. Therefore without negating the world view that one can be attacked by witchcraft, it is possible to address the issue of why the spirits have easy access to you, what makes you or your ***ɔkra*** vulnerable. This then becomes a legitimate investigation with hope for removing the vulnerabilities and strengthening personality. Likewise, drug therapy becomes a way of aiding an ailing body that has been attacked.

Apart from traditional religion, the main religions in Ghana are Christianity and Islam. It is important to understand the belief systems and their contexts in order to provide mental health care. The rich heritage of prayer and support, forgiveness for guilt and for dealing with trauma, the possibility of changing one's mind or being transformed can all be annexed for healing. However it is important to be sensitive to individual and idiosyncratic beliefs and practices within a religion (Lothstein, 2002). Often this is what needs to be explored in relation to the general tenets of the religion. All this should impact the way mental health professionals are trained in Ghana.

Case Vignette

A 45 year-old Christian man with a diagnosis of mixed anxiety depression disorder (ICD10) was referred for therapy. He had seen a psychiatrist earlier but had refused medication because he attributed his symptoms to a "spiritual attack". He had somatic symptoms e.g. palpitations, headaches, bodily pains, excessive sleepiness and fear of dying and leaving his children uncared for and a depressed affect but had no underlying somatic pathology. His attributions were explored sympathetically in therapy and it turned out that he felt vulnerable to such attacks from some evil people in his family because of guilt over his cousin's death. He had informed his cousin of some negative behaviours of his wife and he had exclaimed "This woman will kill me" The cousin died a few months later and he felt the stress of the information he had given him had contributed to his death.

On exploring why he felt so vulnerable to evil attacks despite his faith in God's ability to protect him, he indicated he was not living his faith and needed to grow in this area. Apparently a prayer group in his church had been helpful to him in the past. He was encouraged to rejoin this group and also worked out a behavioural plan to be more consistent with his church Bible studies. A simple explanation of how psychological events could lead to somatic symptoms was given using the flight or fight response of sympathetic arousal. After discussion, he concluded that since the devil knew how his body worked he could attack him by fanning his "danger signals" so sympathetic arousal could occur. Therapy was construed as an opportunity for him to explore the thoughts and feelings that led to "danger signals". This would remove what the devil was using to attack him. A return to Bible study would encourage him in his bid to grow spiritually and strengthen him against further attacks.

He was willing to come for his therapy sessions thereafter and often expressed relief because he said for the first time in his life, he felt able to talk about issues in his past, present and even future life. Issues of forgiveness of self and others were dealt with in therapy and he gradually felt better. He was able to discontinue therapy after five sessions but came intermittently afterwards to deal with specific issues he wanted to explore. His most significant change was his understanding that he could affect his emotional and physical life positively or negatively through his thoughts, values, beliefs and actions and felt capable to do so himself and with the help of others.

The Way Forward - Impacting Religious Healing

Many Ghanaians receive mental health care mainly from religious sources. There are prayer camps, shrines, spiritualists, individual counselling and prayer from pastors or imams etc. There is a need for collaboration with these sources to ensure good mental health care and the eradication of practises that violate the rights of patients. The Ghana Mental Health Act 2012 has paved the way for regulation of services that are given by such religious institutions and individuals. However there is a need for substantial research and investigation into their practices for effective collaboration. At present such research is ongoing (Ofori-Atta & Baning, 2012). Collaboration could be in the area of expanding spiritual practitioners' conceptualizations of psychopathology to include the physical, emotional, cognitive as well as effective drug therapy.

The Way Forward -Training Of Mental Health Professionals

Even in the Euro-American tradition, the importance of religious life in the genesis and treatment of mental illness is now acknowledged. The Accreditation Council for Graduate Medical Education (ACGME) of the American Medical Association requires didactic and clinical instruction on religion and spirituality in psychiatric care. Blass (2007) outlined noteworthy assessment and treatment framework for teaching psychiatry residents how to give service to religious patients. In the Ghanaian and African context, such training is even more imperative considering the importance of spirituality in daily life. In the training of clinical psychologists in the University of Ghana, their psychopathology and psychotherapy courses include topics on traditional conceptualisations of psychopathology and treatment. This could be further expanded as research into religious healing of psychopathology provides increasing evidence to support its healing claims. Also, a basic understanding of traditional religion, Christianity and Islam is also necessary for all mental health professionals in Ghana.

References

Acocella, J. (2000). The Empty Couch: What is lost when psychiatry turns to drugs? *The New Yorker,* May 8.

Anandarajah, G. & Hight, E. (2001). Spirituality and medical practice: Using the HOPE questions as a practical tool for spiritual assessment. *American Family Physician*, 63: 81-89.

Assimeng, M., (1989). *Religion and Social Change in West Africa.* Accra: Ghana Universities Press.

Blass, D.M., (2007). A pragmatic approach to teaching psychiatric residents the assessment and treatment of religious patients. *Academic Psychiatry,* 31:25-31.

Danquah, J.B (1968). Akan Doctrine of God. In: H.M. Feinberg; *African Historical Studies;* Vol 2, No. 1 (1969), pp. 149 – 151. Boston University African Studies Center. Available at:http://www.jstor.org/stable/216335.

Dein, S. (2010). Religion, spirituality and mental health: Theoretical and clinical perspectives. *Psychiatric Times,* 27 no1 No. 1. Available at: http://www.psychiatrictimes.com/articles/religion-spirituality-and-mental-health. [Accessed 19 December 2013].

Dopamu, A. (1985). Health and healing with traditional African religious context. *Orita,* 17: 66-80.

Ferrell, B.R. (2013) Belief in Miracles in Terminal Illness. Medscape, Psychiatry and Mental Health. (March 13) Available at: http://www.medscape.com/viewarticle/780343. [Accessed 9 December 2013].

Field, M.J. (1960). Search for security: An ethno-psychiatric study of rural Ghana. London: Faber & Faber.

Fisher, R. (1998) *West Africa Religious Traditions: Focus on the Akan of Ghana*. Maryknoll.

Frank, J.D., (1973). ***Persuasion and Healing***. New York, Schocken Books, Johns Hopkins University Press.

Lawrence, R.M. & Duggal, A. (2001). Spirituality in psychiatric education and training. *Journal of the Royal Society of Medicine*. 94: 303-305.

Lothstein, L.M. (2002). Book Forum: Handbook of Psychotherapy and Religious Diversity. American *Journal of Psychiatry*, 159: 883-885.

Mbiti, J. S. (1975). *An introduction to African Religion*, London, Heinemann.

Ofori-Atta A.L. & Banning F. (2012). Joining forces; integrating psychotropic medications into the care of people with mental disorders in a prayer camp in Ghana. Perse Comm.

Ofori-Atta A L. & Linden, W. (1995). The effect of social change on causal beliefs of mental disorders and treatment preferences in Ghana. *Social Science and Medicine,* 40 (9) 1231-1242.

Sefa-Dedeh, A., (2001). Psychotherapy and Religion: The Significance of Religious Beliefs and Traditions for Therapy in Ghana, Unpublished paper presented at the Convention of Black Psychiatrists, Ghana.

Twumasi, P. A., (1975). Medical Systems in Ghana. A Study of Medical Sociology. Tema: Ghana Publishing Corporation.

Chapter 7

The state of autism in Ghana: A focus on cultural understanding and challenges in the Ghanaian setting

Joana Salifu and C.Charles Mate-Kole

Introduction

Autism is a lifelong neuro-developmental disability that presents with impairments in social skills, verbal and nonverbal communication, repetitive behaviours and unusual interests (American Psychological Association, APA, 2000). People with autism do not usually participate in pretend play; they have difficulties initiating social interactions, and they engage in self-stimulatory behaviours such as hand flapping, making unusual noises, rocking from side to side and toe-walking (Centres for Disease Control, CDC, 2007). These impairments may range from severe to subtle symptoms of social and communication deficits (Caronna, Milunsky, & Tager-Flusberg, 2008).

Autism was first described by Leo Kanner in 1943. In his original paper, *Autistics Disturbances of Affective Contact*, Kanner described 11 children who had a rare syndrome of "extreme autistic aloneness". Children described by Kanner exhibited severe language impairment, social isolation, instances of sameness, and motor stereotypies (Kanner, 1943). Kanner named the syndrome "infantile autism" because he discovered that the children in his study started exhibiting symptoms in the early ages, precisely before the age of 36 months.

Hans Asperger in 1944 also described a group of children with similar symptoms. The difference between Kanner's autism and Asperger's lies in the degree of severity. Asperger's definition was far broader than Kanner's and included children with higher functioning and intact language abilities (Anthony, 2009). Autism is classified under a broader diagnostic category of pervasive developmental disorders (PDD; Diagnostic and Statistical Manual of Mental Disorders

– Fourth Edition, Text Revision; (DSM-IV-TR – American Psychiatric Association, APA, 2002). Autism is now viewed as a 'spectrum' presenting on a continuum from mild to severe handicap.

Autism Spectrum Disorder (ASD) is presently used to classify autism, Asperger's disorder and other non-specified disorders. Asperger's syndrome is used to describe individuals with milder form of autistic disorder. These individuals may have relatively normal intelligence levels and intact language abilities or minimal language delays but usually have impaired social skills. Individuals with 'classic autism' are non-verbal and present symptoms of severe cognitive impairment, as well as severe motor stereotypic and disruptive behaviours (Caronna et al., 2008).

Besides behavioural deficits, individuals with autism present with cognitive deficits. Some of the cognitive deficits include perceptual problems, information processing difficulties, memory impairment, deficits in executive function and attention, and in acquisition of theory of mind (this provides the explanation for impairment in social reciprocity and communication) (Frith, 1989; Hill, 2004a; Tager-Flusberg, 2007). Deficits in central coherence explain the tendency for autistic individuals to lack focus on local features of the environment (Jolliffe & Baron-Cohen, 1999).

One of the most prominent features of autism is executive function deficits which have profound impact on the autistic individual (Ozonoff, Pennington, & Rogers, 1991). Executive function is traditionally used as an umbrella term for functions such as planning, working memory, impulse control, inhibition, and shifting set, as well as the initiation and monitoring of one's action (Hill, 2004a; Happe, Booth, Charlton, & Hughes, 2006; Hill, 2004b; Hughes, 1998).

The theory of executive function deficit can be used to address behavioural problems such as a need for sameness, a strong liking for repetitive behaviours, lack of impulse control, difficulty initiating new non-routine actions and difficulty switching between tasks (Hill, 2004a; Lopez, Lincoln, Ozonoff, & Lai, 2005; Rajendran & Mitchell, 2007). Besides the cognitive deficits, studies have consistently found deficits in adaptive behaviour in autism (Bolte & Pouska, 2002; Liss et al., 2001). Adaptive behaviours are everyday living skills that people use to adjust to situations in their environment (Liss et al., 2001). The dimension of adaptive skills includes motor, communication, socialization, home living and community living skills, self-care and functional academic skills. These behaviours are known to promote independence, social adjustment and quality of life (Matson, Mayville, & Laud, 2003). Additionally, adaptive behaviours allow people to substitute disruptive behaviours with constructive ones (Gillham, Carter, Volkmar, & Sparrow, 2000).

Prevalence

The prevalence of autism is reported in the range between 1 to 21.1 per 10 ,000 children (World Health Organization; WHO, 2003). In the United States, it is estimated that 1 in every 150 people suffer from autism (CDC, 2007). Studies in Europe and Scandinavia report as many as 12 in 10,000 children (Baird, Simonoff, Pickles, et al., 2006; Kadesjo, Gillberg, & Hagberg, 1999). Recent epidemiological studies in the USA and Great Britain have reported a significant increase in ASD (Caronna et al., 2008). The increase in prevalence has been attributed in part to the broadening of diagnostic classification that includes individuals with relative milder symptoms, although real increase has also been suggested (Caronna et al., 2008). In terms of gender variation, autism is three to four times more common in males than in females (Hill, 2004a; Rutter, 2003).

In Ghana, there is insufficient data and there is no separate category for autism (Anthony, 2009). Students with autism are included in the categories, "Intellectual Disability" (ID) or "Mental Handicap/Mentally Handicapped" (MH) for educational purposes. ID or MH is narrowly defined as having sub-average intelligence (Anthony, 2009). In 2005, the Ghana Education Service reported a total of 955 students enrolled in government-run special schools for the "Mentally Handicapped" (Ministry of Education, Sports and Science, MoESS, 2005). In 2008, MoESS reported that of the 14,596 students screened for impairment, 101 were "clinically assessed" as having "Intellectual Disability" or "Mental Handicap/Mentally Handicapped". The figure reported by MoESS only accounts for students who are enrolled in public schools. This account may underestimate the actual number of children with disabilities in Ghana, given that children who are not enrolled in school were not included. Additionally, these figures do not provide information specifically about the prevalence of autism in Ghana.

In an external epidemiological survey of Special Educational Needs (SEN) (Boro, Grigorenko, Hart, Jarvin, & Kwadade, 2006), a screening instrument was administered to 551 caregivers, siblings and teachers of children throughout Ghana. Some questions were asked that relate to autism. The finding indicated that 3.1 percent of respondents indicated 'yes' to the label "developmental delay or autism" and 3.9 percent responded 'yes' to the label "mental retardation or mental handicap". Although autism forms part of a broader developmental disorder, autism is a unique disorder. Thus, there is the need for it to be recognised as a unique disorder.

Major theoretical perspectives and related studies

Autism was initially theorized by Bruno Bettelheim (Caronna et al., 2008) to be caused by "refrigerated mothers" raising children in a non-stimulating environment. Bettelheim hypothesized that the non-stimulating environment resulted in damage to the children's social, language and general development. Bettelheim's theory has been refuted due to lack of empirical evidence. To date, the main cause of autism remains unclear, although genetic and brain abnormalities have been implicated (Caronna et al., 2008).

Regarding cognitive deficits, specifically executive function, two significant theories were propounded; the *frontal lobe hypothesis* (Baddeley & Wilson, 1988; Stuss & Benson, 1983) and the *supervisory system model* (Norman & Shallice, 1980) to explain executive function deficits in autism. The frontal lobe is known for its role in high-level modulation of lower-level processes supported by posterior brain regions (Gilbert & Burgess, 2008). It sends and receives projections from virtually all major sensory and motor cortical systems, with access to highly processed multi-modal sensory information represented in higher-order sensory regions. Interconnections between the prefrontal cortex (PFC) and sub-cortical structures, such as the basal ganglia have been identified. Thus, the PFC is well placed to integrate diverse, high-level representations, and to exert control over various brain systems. The patterns of activity within PFC represent current behavioural context and/or current goals and intentions (Gilbert & Burgess, 2008).

The involvement of the frontal lobe in executive function was first suggested by Damasio and Maurer (1978) who observed some similarities between deficit patterns in individuals with autism and those with frontal lobe injuries. Executive functions such as set-shifting, inhibition of prepotent responses, self-monitoring and planning are thought to be associated with the functions of the frontal lobes, precisely the pre-frontal cortex (Gilbert & Burgess, 2008; Ozonoff et al., 2004; Pennington & Ozonoff, 1996). As a result, deficits in executive functioning are thought to result from frontal lobe damage and associated areas such as the basal ganglia and the limbic system (Stuss & Knight, 2002). Impulsivity, perseveration and a failure to pursue goals over long periods of time have been found to be amongst the most common difficulties reported after frontal lobe damage, which are also present in autistic individuals. Other evidence comes from the frontal lobe involvement in functional imaging (Baron-Cohen et al., 1999; Gilbert & Burgess, 2008; Luna et al., 2002; Minshew, Luna, & Sweeney, 1999) and neuropathological investigations (Casanova, Buxhoeveden, Switala, & Roy, 2002).

Among autistic individuals, it has been noted that most of the tasks that measure executive functions in which individuals show deficits are mediated by the frontal lobes (Stuff, 2009). Studies have reported clinical similarities between individuals with autism and adults with frontal lesions (Damasio & Maurer, 1978; Gilbert & Burgess, 2008; Hughes, 1998). This suggests that executive function deficits in autism may result from deficits in the frontal lobes.

The supervisory system model conceptualized executive function in terms of two pivotal components within a selection-for-action system. These components include the contention scheduling and the supervisory attentional system. The contention scheduler is known to mediate the effect of the environment when automatic or routine actions are selected. When the contention scheduling component is triggered, it controls the mutual inhibition of competing actions (since many actions may be triggered at once) so that the most appropriate course of action would be selected (Norman & Shallice, 1980; Bell, 2010).

The two systems are likened to thoughts or action schemas that govern behaviour (Gilbert & Burgess, 2008). These schemas are activated in two ways. First, they could be triggered by events in one's environment. Environmental triggering of schemas (contention scheduler) can be sufficient to accomplish appropriate behaviour in routine situations that involve well-learned links between particular events in our environment and particular ways of behaving.

In situations where the contending scheduler is not sufficient due to novel situations, damage to the supervisory system may lead to excessive behavioural rigidity (Gilbert & Burgess, 2008). In other situations where there is a reduction in supervisory input it may lead to the triggering of inappropriate behaviour by salient objects in the environment, leading to excessive distractibility. Thus, damage to the supervisory system could explain excessive rigidity and distractibility, both of which have been reported to occur following damage to the frontal lobes (Gilbert & Burgess, 2008).

Neuropsychological studies have shown that particular impairments can lead to deficits in executive functions such as distractibility, planning, inhibition and cognitive flexibility (Bell, 2010; Gurd, 1995; Shallice & Burgess, 1996). The supervisory system model can explain why autistic individuals are good at doing routine tasks but have difficulties performing novel tasks and are unable to inhibit a learned response.

The frontal lobe is also related to adaptive functioning skills which provide explanation to related deficits in adaptive behaviours and executive function in autism. The prefrontal cortex has been shown to be involved in the regulation of social behaviour, emotional reactions, and social discourse (Dennis, 1991; Price, Daffner, Stowe, & Mesulam, 1990; Stuss, 1992). As a result, when there are deficits in executive function, deficits in adaptive behaviours are expected given that the two functions are regulated by the same organ, hence the correlation found between executive functions and adaptive skills (Dawson et al., 2002; Gillotty, Kenworthy, Sirian, Black, & Wagner, 2002; McEvoy, Rogers & Pennington, 1993; Ozonoff & McEvoy, 1994).

In another study, Happe et al. (2006) aimed to map out specific domains of executive function deficits in boys with high functioning autism and Asperger disorder compared to boys with attention deficit and hyperactivity disorder (ADHD) and those with non-pathological conditions. The authors found that among the autism group, older boys performed significantly better than younger boys on six cognitive tasks including fluency, spatial working memory and constructional skills. In comparison to the typically developing individuals, younger autistics made significantly more verbal fluency errors on the fluency tasks and they needed more time on planning. Happe et al. concluded that these deficits persist throughout the life span of the autistic individual (Hill, 2004b; Robinson, Goddard, Dritschel, Wisley, & Howlin, 2009).

As reflected in the earlier review, the majority of studies conducted on autism and its related cognitive deficits were carried out in the countries outside Africa. To date, and to our knowledge, only one study (Salifu, 2011) has been done in the Ghanaian setting. As a result, little is known about cognitive deficits among individuals with autism in Ghana. Knowledge obtained from such studies which could have assisted in the management of individuals with autism is thus lacking.

Additionally, some studies on the relationship between executive function and age in autism have found significant age differences (Happe et al., 2006; Ozonoff and Jensen, 1999; Robinson et al., 2009) although other studies did not report such deficits (Ozonoff & McEvoy's, 1994; Ozonoff et al., 2004). Most of these studies employed high-functioning individuals, neglecting the low-functioning individuals who form the majority of autistic individuals. Thus, it is unclear whether deficits progress with age or not in low functioning autistic individuals.

Theoretical and empirical evidence and its relevance to the Ghanaian concepts

The cultural views of autism in general and how executive function deficits affect individuals with autism in Ghana warrant comments. This review is of importance because some of the negative cultural beliefs that surround autism can be explained by the resulting deficits in executive function and adaptive skill.

In Ghana, there is a cultural misunderstanding surrounding autism as a disorder as well as the causes of autism. Anthony (2009) reported that the perceived causes of autism in Ghana are complex and vary widely over time and circumstances. Some people seem to turn to biomedical explanations while others look to spiritual forces. From a biomedical perspective, autism is perceived to be caused by severe illnesses, high fever or seizures (typically called 'convulsion') to the child at a young age. Other explanations are focused on blaming the mother of a child with autism. Such explanations include illnesses or accident to the mother while pregnant; a failed abortion attempt by the mother typically involving the ingestion of tonics; a lack of 'maternal effort' during childbirth; and the result of maternal error (mother not being faithful to her husband or mother not having a husband).

From a spiritual perspective, some Ghanaians in Anthony's (2009) study perceived autism to be caused by demons with spiritual powers or through retribution from higher powers. With respect to human factors, autism is believed to be caused by retribution for transgressions committed against someone close to the family with autistic children. This is believed to be done either through directly enacting justice or hiring a spiritual practitioner to do the act on the child or unborn infants. Some other human factors are blamed on jealous rivals, punishment for greed (blood money) or failure to uphold Ghanaian values, and seeking fertility from spirits. Other people also believe that individuals with autism are witches themselves (Anthony, 2009).

We would argue that behaviours of autistic individuals may be due to executive function deficits and deficits in adaptive skills. The key symptoms of autism (deficits in communication, socialization and restricted behaviour) make it difficult for autistic individuals to fit into the Ghanaian culture. The ability to communicate and socialise are highly valued in Ghana. The culture is known for its collectiveness, interdependency and reciprocal obligation to one's community and family (Nukunya, 2003). As a result, the isolation and reclusiveness of autistic children worsen the stigma already held against them. Also, the lack of imaginative play makes it difficult for individuals with autism to engage in activities with other children.

Directions for future research and conclusion

Although executive function and adaptive skills in autism have been well studied in the Western world, little is known about Ghanaian autistic children. Findings from Western culture cannot be generalised to the Ghanaian population due to cultural differences. It is therefore important that appropriate measures that are culturally sensitive to Ghanaian samples are used to examine executive functions in autistic individuals.

It is necessary to establish whether executive function deficits found in the Western world are similar or different from the Ghanaian autistic population. This is important given that a study (Salifu, 2011) on executive function in the Ghanaian context did not find improvement in executive function deficits with age. Further, it is possible that deficits did not improve in the Ghanaian sample due to lack of cognitive training. There are inherent differences in Ghanaian autistic individuals that have not been explored. Of note, in Ghana, interventions developed in the Western world for training in executive functions for autistic individuals are generally used. It is possible that due to lack of information on the Ghanaian autistic sample, such intervention strategies might not be appropriate for Ghanaian individuals. This might be due to differences in the presentation of deficits patterns.

As outlined earlier, it is evident that autism as a disorder has received little attention and it is misunderstood in the Ghanaian setting. Thus, more attention should be focused on the study of autism in Ghana.

Autism needs to be categorised as a distinct disorder - this is necessary in order for studies to be carried out particularly on the prevalence as well as on the nature of the disorder in the Ghanaian setting. It is clear that most cultural misunderstanding about the behaviours of individuals with autism can be explained by theories on cognitive deficits and deficits in adaptive behaviours. However, little psycho-education been done in this regard. The misconceptions about autism in the Ghanaian context can be attributed to lack of awareness and knowledge. Information about the nature of autism, especially with respect to executive function and adaptive behaviour, can help to minimize the misconceptions held by Ghanaians about autism. A better understanding of the condition can improve the care and quality of life of the autistic individual.

References

American Psychiatric Association (2000). *Diagnostic and Statistical Manual of Mental Disorders* (DSM-IV TR, 4th ed. text revision). Washington, DC: American Psychiatric Association.

Anthony, J. H. (2009). *Towards Inclusion: Influences of Culture and Internationalisation on Personhood, Educational Access, Policy and Provision for Students with Autism in Ghana* (Doctoral dissertation). Available at: http://sro.sussex.ac.uk/2347/1/Anthony,_Jane_H..pdf

Baddeley, A. D., & Wilson, B. (1988). Frontal amnesia and the dysexecutive syndrome. *Brain and Cognition*, 7, 212–230.

Baird, G., Simonoff, E., Pickles, A., Chandler, S., Loucas, T., Meldrum, D., & Charman, T. (2006). Prevalence of disorders of the autism spectrum in a population cohort of children in South Thames: The Special Needs and Autism Project (SNAP). *Lancet*, *15*, 179–181.

Baron-Cohen, S., Ring, H., Wheelwright, S., Bullmore, E., Brammer, M., Simmons, A., & Williams, S. (1999). Social intelligence in the normal and autistic brain: An fMRI study. *Journal of Autism and Developmental Disorders*, *34*, 139–150.

Bell, V. (2010). *The executive system and its disorders*. Available at: http://www.cognitivesolutionslc.com/execsysdisorders.pdf.

Bolte, S., & Poustka, F. (2002). The relationship between general cognitive level and adaptive domains in individuals with autism with and without co-morbid mental retardation. *Child Psychiatry and Human Development*, 33, 165–172.

Boro, E., Grigorenko, E., Hart, L., Jarvin, L., & Kwadade, D. D. (2006). *An Overview of the EQUALL-SEN Fall 2005 Epidemiological Survey in Damongo, Koforidua, and Ho Districts: Instruments, Samples, Methods, and Results, Education Quality for All Project (EQUALL)*. Accra, Ghana.

Caronna, E. B., Milunsky, J. M., & Tager-Flusberg, H. (2008). Autism spectrum disorders: Clinical and research frontiers. *Archives of Disorders in Childhood*, *93*, 518–523.

Casanova, M. F., Buxhoeveden, D. P., Switala, A. E., & Roy, E. (2002). Minicolumnar pathology in autism. *Journal of Autism and Developmental Disorders*, *34*, 139–150.

Centers for Disease Control and Prevalence (CDC, 2007). Prevalence of Autism spectrum disorder. Autism and Developmental disabilities monitoring networks, 14 sites, United States, 2002. *MMWR*, *56*, 1–55.

Damasio, A. R., & Maurer, R. G. (1978). A Neurological Model for Childhood Autism. *Archives of Neurology*, *35*, 777–786.

Dawson, G., Carver, L., Meltzoff, A. N., Panagiotides, H., McPartland, J., & Webb, S. J. (2002). Neural correlates of face and object recognition in young children with autism spectrum disorder, developmental delay, and typical development. *Child Development*, *73*, 700–717.

Dennis, M. (1991). Frontal lobe function in childhood and adolescence: A heuristic for assessing attention regulation, executive control, and the intentional states important for social discourse. Special Issue: Developmental consequences of early frontal lobe damage. *Developmental Neuropsychology*, *7*, 327–358.

Fisch, G. S., Simensen, R. J., & Schroer, R. J. (2002). Longitudinal changes in cognitive and adaptive behavior scores in children and adolescents with the Fragile X mutation or autism. *Journal of Autism and Developmental Disorders*, *32*, 107–114.

Frith, U. (1989). *Autism: Explaining the enigma*. Oxford: Blackwell.

Gilbert, S. J., & Burgess, P. W. (2008). Executive Function. *Current Biology*, *18*, 110–114.

Gillham, J. E., Carter, A. S., Volkmar, F. R., & Sparrow, S. S. (2000). Towards a developmental operational definition of autism. *Journal of Autism and Developmental Disorders*, *30*, 269–278.

Gillotty, L., Kenworthy, L., Sirian, L., Black, D. O., & Wagner, A. E. (2002). Adaptive skills and executive function in autism spectrum disorders. *Clinical Neuropsychology*, *8*, 241–248.

Gurd, J. M. (1995). Frontal dissociations: Evidence from Parkinson's disease. *Journal of Neurolinguistics*, *9*, 55–68.

Happe, F., Booth, R., Charlton, R., & Hughes, C. (2006). Executive function deficits in autism spectrum disorders and attention-deficit/hyperactivity disorder: Examining profiles across domains and ages. *Brain and Cognition*, *61*, 25–39.

Hill, E. L. (2004a). Executive dysfunction in autism. *Trends in Cognitive Sciences*, *8*, 26–32.

Hill, E. L. (2004b). Evaluating the theory of executive dysfunction in autism. *Developmental Review*, *24*, 189–233.

Hughes, C. (1998). Executive function in preschoolers: Links with theory of mind and verbal ability. *British Journal of Developmental Psychology*, *16*, 233–253.

Jolliffe, T., & Baron-Cohen, S. (1999). The Strange Stories Test: A replication with high functioning adults with autism or Asperger syndrome. *Journal of Autism and Developmental Disorders*, *29*, 395–404.

Kadesjo B., Gillberg C., & Hagberg B. (1999). Autism and Asperger syndrome in seven year-old children: A total population study. *Journal of Autism and Developmental Disorders*, *29*, 327–331.

Kanner, L. (1943). Autistic disturbances of affective contact. *Nervous Child*, 2, 217–250.

Liss, M., Fein, D., Allen, D., Dunn, M., Feinstein, C., Morris, R., & Rapin, I. (2001). Executive Functioning in High-functioning Children with Autism. *Journal of Child Psychology and Psychiatry*, *42*, 261–270.

Lopez, B. R., Lincoln, A. J., Ozonoff, S., & Lai, Z. (2005). Examining the relationship executive functions and restricted, repetitive symptoms of autistic disorder. *Journal of Autism and Developmental Disorders*, *35*, 445–461.

Luna, B., Minshew, N. J, Garver, K. E., Lazar, N. A., Thulborn, K. R., Eddy, W. F., & Sweeney, J. A. (2002). Neocortical system abnormalities in autism: An fMRI study of spatial working memory. *Neurology*, *59*, 834–840.

Matson, J. L., Mayville, S. B., & Laud, R. B. (2003). A system of assessment for adaptive behavior, social skills, behavioural function, medication side-effects, and psychiatric disorders. *Research in Developmental Disabilities*, *24*, 75–81.

McEvoy, R. E., Rogers, S. J., & Pennington, B. F. (1993). Executive function and social communication deficits in young autistic children. *Journal of Child Psychology and Psychiatry*, *34*, 563–578

Ministry of Education Sports & Science (MoESS) (2005). *Preliminary Education Sector Performance Report,* Accra: Republic of Ghana.

Minshew, M. J., Luna, B., & Sweeney, J. A. (1999). Oculomotor evidence for neocortical systems but not cerebellar dysfunction in autism. *Journal of Autism and Developmental Disorders*, *34*, 139–150.

Norman, D. A., & Shallice, T. (1980). Attention to action: Willed and automatic control of behavior. *Current biology*, *18*, 110–114.

Nukunya, G. K. (2003). *Tradition and Change in Ghana: an Introduction to Sociology,* (2nd Edition). Accra: Ghana Universities Press.

Ozonoff, S., & Jensen, J. (1999). Brief report: Specific executive function profiles in three neurodevelopmental disorders. *Journal of Autism and Developmental Disorders*, *29*, 171–177.

Ozonoff, S., & McEvoy, R. E. (1994). A longitudinal study of executive function and theory of mind development in autism. *Development and Psychopathology*, 6, 415–431.

Ozonoff, S., Cook, I., Coon, H., Dawson, G., Joseph, M. R., Klin, A., . . . & Wrathall, D. (2004). Performance on Cambridge Neuropsychological Test Automated Battery Subtests Sensitive to Frontal Lobe Function in People with Autistic Disorder: Evidence from the Collaborative Programs of Excellence in Autism Network. *Journal of Autism and Developmental Disorders*, *34*, 139–150.

Ozonoff, S., Pennington, B. F., & Rogers, S. J. (1991). Executive function deficits in high-functioning autistic individuals: Relationship to theory of mind. *Journal of Child Psychology and Psychiatry*, 32, 1081–1105.

Pennington, B. F., & Ozonoff, S. (1996). Executive functions and developmental psychopathologies. *Journal of Child Psychology and Psychiatry*, *37*, 51–87.

Price, B. H., Daffner, K. R., Stowe, R. M., & Mesulam, M. M. (1990). The compartmental learning disabilities of early frontal lobe damage. *Journal of Autism and Developmental Disorders*, *34*, 139–150.

Rajendran, G., & Mitchell, P. (2007). Cognitive theories of Autism. *Developmental Review*, 27, 224–260.

Robinson, S., Goddard, L., Dritschel, B., Wisley, M., & Howlin, P. (2009). Executive functions in children with Autism Spectrum Disorders. *Brain and Cognition*, *71*, 362–368

Rutter, M. (2003). Introduction: Autism–the challenge ahead. In: G. Bock, & J. Goode (Eds.), *Autism: Neural basis and treatment possibilities* (pp. 1–9). Chichester: Wiley.

Salifu, J. (2011). *Executive function deficit in autistic individuals in Ghana* (Unpublished master's thesis). University of Ghana, Legon.

Shallice, T., & Burgess, P. (1996). The domain of supervisory processes and temporal organization of behavior. *Philosophical Transactions of the Royal Society of London*, *351*, 1405–1412.

Stuff, N. (2009). *Executive functions in ASD*. Retrieved from www.noustuff.wordpress.com/2009/11/06/.

Stuss, D. T., & Benson, D. F. (1983). The frontal lobes. In: D. T. Stuss, & R. T. Knight (Eds.), *Principles of frontal lobe function* (pp. 408–427). Oxford: Oxford University Press.

Stuss, D. T., & Knight, R. T. (2002). *Principles of frontal lobe function*. Oxford: Oxford University Press.

Stuss, D. T. (1992). Biological and psychological development of executive functions. *Brain and Cognition*, 20, 8–23.

Tager-Flusberg, H. (2007). Evaluating the Theory-of-mind hypothesis of Autism. *Current Directions in Psychological Science*, 6, 311–315.

World Health Organization (2003). *The World Health Report, 2003: Shaping the future*. Geneva: WHO.

Chapter 8

Substance Use Disorders in Ghana

J. B. Asare and Akua Afriyie Addae

Introduction

Historically, human beings have used psychoactive substances for various reasons including medicinal, cultural/ religious and recreational purposes. However, the last century, which brought enhanced scientific and pharmacological advancement, resulted in the manufacture of synthetic and semi-synthetic drugs which were more potent, caused dependency and unfortunately became the preferred substances of use, particularly by the youth.

Several reasons for the increased abuse of drugs have been postulated. The reasons include availability, experimentation, peer group influences, ignorance about the efficacy of the drug used and stresses of everyday life.

The World Health Organization (WHO 2012) reports that globally, at least 15.3 million persons have substance use disorders. Alcohol alone results in 2.5 million deaths (of which 320,000 are between ages 15 and 29 years) each year and is the world's third largest risk factor for premature mortality, disability and loss of health. It also estimates that 155 to 250 million people, or 3.5% to 5.7% of the world's population aged 15-64, use other psychoactive substances such as cannabis, amphetamines, cocaine, opioids, and non-prescribed psychoactive prescription medication with cannabis being the commonest (129 -190 million).

Substance abuse and drug trafficking have become a problem all over the world. Whereas we have our own problems in dealing with socially accepted substances like alcohol and tobacco, in recent times Ghana is being confronted with the trafficking of drugs like cannabis, cocaine, heroin, amphetamine type stimulants and precursor chemicals. Ghana has been designated a transit country and as a rule some of the narcotic and psychotropic substances being trafficked remain in the country to be used. It is sad to observe on missions to many African countries conducted by the International Narcotics Control Board (of which the first author was a member), that many African countries do not have adequate controls for narcotics or for the precursors used in their manufacture (for example acetic anhydride or vinegar added to an opium base which is used to produce heroin or potassium permanganate used to prepare cocaine). Consequently, the traffickers are capitalizing on the weaknesses of the control systems to divert and traffic in these substances.

Drug traffickers are increasingly using West African countries along the Gulf of Guinea for smuggling cocaine from Latin America into Europe and to a lesser extent to America. This is evidenced by the volume of seizures effected in this sub-region (International Narcotic Control Board (INCB, 2006).

Drug production, distribution and consumption are associated with violence, gangs, theft, corruption and abuse of public authority. Armed conflicts in many parts of Africa have been fought by youth who have been misguided to use drugs to commit more atrocities than we can imagine.

The increase in the prevalence of HIV/AIDS infection globally is a matter of concern with 69 percent of the world's HIV/AIDS population living in sub-Saharan Africa (WHO, 2012). In Ghana, although there is reduced prevalence of HIV/AIDS, the prevalence may have been further decreased had there not been the increased use of drugs whose association with injection and risky sexual behaviour has been recognized as a risk factor for the spread of the disease. In this regard, it is very necessary that concerted efforts among countries be made for the effective management of the problem of drug abuse.

Types of substances commonly abused in Ghana

For the purposes of this paper, drug will apply to substances that affect the functions of the brain which can manifest in abnormalities in behavioural, perceptual and thinking processes. The common drugs of abuse include alcohol, tobacco, cannabis, cocaine, heroin, amphetamine and amphetamine-type stimulants, sedative-hypnotics such as pethidine and morphine and other prescribed drugs. (Asare, 2009).

Alcohol is the most commonly abused substance in our environment (Asare, 1999) with prevalence of 23.5 percent among the youth (WHO, 2011; Dennis-Antwi, et al, 2003). A WHO (2011) statistic indicates that the per capita recorded alcohol consumption among adults of 15 years and above in Ghana, increased from 0.44 litres in 1996 to 1.5 litres in 2005, while that of unrecorded consumption was estimated at 1.5 litres. The national prevalence of alcohol use disorders among the same age group was estimated at 1.43 percent and 0.16 percent for males and females respectively. Its abuse is largely linked with the socio-cultural life of Ghanaians, ignorance of its effects and corporate advertisement. In Ghana, as is in most African countries, people with alcohol related problems are treated mainly in general hospitals. For example in South Africa, it is estimated that 30 percent of general hospital admissions are directly or indirectly related to alcohol (Hammond, 2004).

Cannabis is the main narcotic drug of abuse in Ghana and the world with a prevalence rate of 2.6 to 9 percent - about 119 million to 224 million people (INCB, 2006). Its cultivation is on the increase and evidence available indicates that Afghanistan is the world's largest global producer of cannabis resins, with Morocco producing most of Europe's cannabis (United Nations Office on Drugs and Crime-UNODC, 2012). Local names includes wee/weed, Marijuana, Ganja, Indian Hemp, Timber, Rolls, Stuff, ***Taaba, Ntampe, Abonsam tawa, Abele, Ahabanmono, Gari, Popoje, and Sundu*** (Dennis-Antwi et al., 2003).

Cannabis is known to be a contributory factor to the occurrence of schizophrenic-like psychosis. The plant grows wild throughout most tropical and temperate regions of the world. Prior to the production of synthetic fibre, the cannabis plant was cultivated for the tough fibre of its stem. The producers of cannabis are small scale farmers while the distributors are young people from urban centres. The consumers represent the youth and adults from all the different strata of the economic ladder. The traffickers are people who are well established with connections to power. The production of cannabis may be related to unemployment and the fact that it is a profitable activity with better economic reward than traditional crops.

Delta-9 Tetrahydrocannabinol (THC) is believed to be responsible for most of the psychoactive effects of cannabis. Three illicit drugs that are produced from cannabis are Marijuana, hashish and cannabis oil. Marijuana comes from the leaves and flowering tops of the cannabis plant that are dried to produce a tobacco-like substance that is smoked. Hashish consists of THC-rich resinous material of the cannabis plant which is collected, dried and then compressed into balls, cakes, or cookie-like sheets. Pieces are then broken off, placed in pipes and smoked. Marijuana contains known toxins and cancer causing chemicals. Some of the effects of marijuana use include palpitations, reddening of the eyes, impaired concentration and hunger. Hallucinations, fantasies and schizophrenic-like symptoms have been reported. Cannabis use in Ghana has been associated with the return of our soldiers who fought in Burma and India during the second war (Asuni, 1992; DuToit (1980) cited in Affinnih, 1999). However, it started to be used on a wider scale in the permissive 1960s.

Cocaine is the most potent stimulant of natural origin. It is extracted from the coca plant (Erythroxylum coca), which is indigenous to the Andean highlands of South America. Illicit cocaine is usually distributed as a white crystalline powder. The powder, usually cocaine hydrochloride, is often snorted or dissolved and injected. ***Crack cocaine,*** which is cocaine mixed with baking soda to increase its quantity is also available in Ghana. It is smoked in pipes, having been prepared into a rock-like substance. Local names apart from crack includes, white powder, energy generator, crazy, Maggie powder, snow, coke, Deck, white lady, fire on the mountain, *Soroabofo, Aweabonsonsa, Buu*. (Dennis-Antwi et al., 2003).

When cocaine is used, a pleasurable state of well-being, relief from fatigue, increased mental alertness, increased physical strength, reduction of hunger and indifference to pain are achieved. Cocaine effects are immediate but short lived. Large doses can lead to paranoia and tactile hallucinations, particularly, feeling as if insects are crawling on the body. A state similar to paranoid schizophrenia may be induced by chronic use. Cocaine abuse surfaced in Ghana in the mid-eighties and its use continues to increase due to its availability. It is an expensive drug which is related to crime on the part of users who need more money to sustain the habit.

Amphetamine Type Stimulants (ATS) are stimulants under international control. They were initially used for Attention Deficit Hyperactivity Disorder (ADHD) and Narcolepsy. Amphetamine type stimulants are not imported into Ghana.

Opiates belong to the large biosynthetic group of alkaloids and are so named because they are naturally occurring alkaloids found in the opium poppy. The major psychoactive opiates are morphine, codeine, thebaine, papaverine and noscapine. Opiates are known to suppress pain response. The effects include general central nervous system depression, reducing pain perception, reducing fear, lessening of inhibitions and elevation of mood. ***Heroin*** is semi-synthetic opiate prepared from opium base and acetic anhydride. Commonly called Brown sugar, Vigo, *Zimblim, Abibe, Para, Ape* and Figure, (Dennis Antwi et al.,.2003) heroin use surfaced in the mid-eighties in Ghana. It comes to Ghana through East Africa, Ethiopia and the United Arab Emirates from South East Asian countries, on its way to Europe and North America. Heroin dependency causes severe withdrawal symptoms when the user abstains. The withdrawal symptoms include pains in the joints, shivering, nasal discharge and lacrimation, diarrhea, abdominal cramps and vomiting.

Heroin is obtained from the opium plant which is not grown in Africa. Its use is however spreading to many African countries. The most worrying aspect is its injection use which is contributing to the spread of HIV/AIDS infection. According to studies done in Kenya, Nigeria and South Africa, prevalence of intravenous drug use appears higher than commonly believed. (Asare & Wellington, 2004). The WHO study in Nairobi city revealed a high number of heroin abusers injecting the drug intravenously. In Lagos, a study carried out in 2000 found that the HIV prevalence rate among heroin and cocaine Street users was almost twice as high as among non drug users (9.8 percent for the former as compared with 5.4 percent for the latter).

Pethidine and Morphine are two common opiates often abused by patients and health personnel who have access to them. Invariably patients are introduced to the substances when they are treated legitimately for severe pain for a period but continue to self-medicate. Some people who are introduced to them become dependent on them because of unprofessional medical practice, weak logistical control, and lack of adequate control systems in hospitals and pharmacies. Withdrawal symptoms and effects are similar to heroin.

Sedative–hypnotics include barbiturates and benzodiazepines. These are abused in large quantities in Ghana. Benzodiazepam is commonly prescribed as sleeping tablets. These drugs are not properly regulated, are very addictive, cause dependency and can be found on sale across the counter in many African countries. Continued use leads to dependency, poor sleep habits and sleep disorders etc.

Volatile substances are inhalable vapours from a number of substances which produce rapid psychoactive effects. Commonly abused products include glue, cleansing fluids, lighter fuels, nail polish remover, paint thinners and aerosol products.

Many African countries have reported the abuse of volatile substances particularly by the youth. This leads to lowered oxygen levels in the brain and disinhibition. The effect is similar to alcohol intoxication but is short lived. Users often feel dizzy, have slurred speech, stagger and have double vision. Some can hallucinate as they become delirious. Prolonged use can lead to brain damage as well as damage to the kidneys and the liver. The abuse of volatile substances in Ghana is not on a wide scale (Dennis-Antwi et al, 2003). We should look out for the victims of abuse of volatile substances without publicizing it, so as not to spread its use out of curiosity.

Lysergic Acid Diethylamide (LSD) was originally derived from fungus that affects grasses and cereal grain and it is manufactured illegally. LSD produces changes in perception ranging from illusions to full scale hallucinations. There is a subjective feeling of increased mental activity, altered body image and changes in the sense of time and place. Psychotic reactions with confusion states may occur. Flashbacks are often common. LSD is abused in some African countries but rarely in Ghana. Apart from South Africa, where significant quantities of synthetic drugs, notably methaqualone (Mandrax) continue to be illicitly manufactured and abused by the local population, there is little information on the abuse of these substances elsewhere in Africa.

MDMA (Ecstasy) is smuggled into South Africa from Europe by air freight and parcel post. (INCB, 2012).

Assessment and essential treatment elements of substance abuse

1. General psychiatric assessment including family history of drug use and mental state examination should be made.
2. Ascertain drug history –types of drugs used, frequency and motivation for their use.
3. Thorough physical examination, including inspection of the skin for injection drug use, systemic examination and neurological examination should be undertaken.
4. Find out if there were brushes with the law particularly with respect to antisocial activities.
5. Administration of standardized tests to identify the type of drugs abused and severity or level of abuse. These include Alcohol Use Disorder Identification Test (AUDIT), Michigan Alcoholism Screening Test (MAST), CAGE (Cut-down; Annoyed; Guilty; Eye-Opener). T-ACE (Tolerance, Annoyed, Cut-down, Eye-Opener), TWEAK (Tolerance, Worried, Eye-Opener, Amnesia, K/Cut-Down) and Addiction Severity Index (ASI).Work needs to be done in the translation and standardization of these measures into common local dialects.
6. Treatment history should be obtained (if any).
7. Formulate care plan which should include Pharmacological and psychosocial interventions.
8. Management of withdrawal effects and co-morbidities essential for safety of patient.
9. Relapse prevention.

Risk and protective factors of substance abuse

Risk factors make one vulnerable to diseases or increase the likelihood that one will engage in unhealthy behaviour" (such as drug use, violence, suicide or early sexual activity) while protective factors help buffer against diseases and other unhealthy behaviours"

Risk and protective factors of substance abuse could be internal (personal) or external (environmental). Thus, personal factors such as self-esteem, personality characteristics, gender and other genetic and personal characteristics serve as risk or protective factors. For instance several studies have shown that males are more likely to use drugs than females Individuals with certain temperaments such as a tendency towards irritability and aggression may be at risk for substance abuse. In addition, mental disorders such as depression, anxiety, post-traumatic stress disorder, ADHD and conduct disorder have been linked with substance use disorder in adolescents. (Affinnih, 1999; Atwoli, 2011; Dennis-Antwi et al, 2003; Doku, Kivusi, Ita & Rimpela, 2012).

External factors that put people at risk or protect them against substance abuse include interpersonal factors and other larger environmental characteristics. For instance social cognitive/learning theory suggests that people learn about substance abuse from significant role models such as parents, peers or close friends through processes of imitation and social reinforcement. The norms of the group or the community people belong to, their beliefs and expectations all can be risk or protective factors. Among adolescents for instance, it has been found that those whose parents and other family members use drugs or have positive attitudes towards drugs are also at risk of abusing drugs (Atwoli et al, 2011; Dennis-Antwi, et al, 2003; Wellington, 2006). Another strong risk factor is the association with peers who engage in risky behaviours like substance abuse. In fact, a number of studies have found peer influence to be a stronger predictor of adolescent substance abuse than parental influences (Atwoli et al, 2011; Bahr, Hoffman & Yang, 2005; Dennis-Antwi et al, 2003; Wellington, 2005). These family members and peers serve as negative role models.

The quality of parental care is also a predictor of adolescent substance abuse. A poor parent-child relationship, inconsistent parental monitoring and supervision have been found to be associated with higher risk of adolescent substance abuse (Clark, Belarare & Abell, 2012). Conflicts at home and with peers, divorce, death of loved ones, unemployment, and poor academic achievement are other risk factors of adolescent substance abuse. Other risk factors are living in neighbourhoods where drugs are readily available and cultures that have positive attitudes towards drug use. In a survey of 4,185 JSS students aged 13-15, Wellington (2006) found that 34.3 percent of the participants reported buying cigarettes in a store while 54.3 percent reported buying cigarettes in a store and not being refused purchase because of their age. Even though there is a ban on advertisement of tobacco in Ghana, adverts on TV and radio continually extol the "virtues" of alcohol. Studies have shown that more exposure to adverts promoting alcohol among teens is linked to higher drinking levels.

External protective factors of adolescent substance abuse include having families and living in communities that have zero tolerance for drugs. Others are healthy parent-child relationship, consistent parental monitoring and supervision (Hawkins, Catano & Miller, 1992). Another important factor that has been found to protect adolescents is religiosity/spirituality (Kovacs, Franciska, & Fitzpatrick, 2011; Mason, Dean, Kelly, & Crowe, 2009). Involvement in religious activities like prayer and other church activities and belief in God (Supreme Being) provide people with motivation for abstinence.

Treatment

Treatment of substance use disorders can be done using individual approaches or a combination of individual and group approaches.

Pharmacological management of withdrawal

Most developing countries are encouraging the use of psychotropic drugs for short term withdrawal of drugs including narcotics. The use of methadone for withdrawal from heroin for instance is expensive and problematic in terms of causing dependency. This is therefore being discouraged.

Diazepam given in sliding (or reduced) doses over 5 days can help. The dangers of causing dependency should be remembered. In most cases, it may be useful to give major tranquillizers to sedate the clients to overcome the tendency to abscond due to the urge to use the drug. Intravenous slow infusions concurrent with sedation will help to keep the client in bed during the withdrawal phase. The withdrawal phase can manifest as yawning, headaches, abdominal cramps, nausea, tremors, sweating, diarrhoea, watery eyes, restlessness and perceptual disorders depending on the substance of abuse.

Treating alcohol, cocaine and other addiction sometimes involves a combination of different strategies and a multi-dimensional approach. Below are some of the treatment modalities for addiction.

Self help Groups: The most common self help groups is the 12-step model by Alcoholics Anonymous (AA) (Kinney, 2003). Using the same model for narcotics and other substances, there is now a plethora of self help groups such as narcotic anonymous (NA) nicotine anonymous, and cocaine anonymous (CA) for treating alcohol, narcotic, nicotine and cocaine addictions (Ray & Ksir, 2004; Kinney, 2003). There are a few of these groups in Ghana with AA being the most dominant. There are AA groups that meet at the Accra Psychiatric Hospital and Addictive Disease Unit-Korle Bu Teaching Hospital.

These groups follow a strict religious and medical model of addiction and hold quasi-religious meetings that are designed to bring addicts into the group (See Table 8.1). According to this model, addicts never recover but are always in the process of recovering. They will be addicts for life, even if they never take another drink or drug.

The main criticism of these groups is their appearance like religious cults with roots in an evangelical group called the Oxford group. Further, very few empirical studies have been done to evaluate the success of AA (Ray & Ksir, 2004).

Psychological Interventions: Many psychotherapeutic techniques have been used to treat substance abuse and addiction. Psychotherapy used in combination with other treatment approaches (especially pharmacological treatment and the 12-steps) have been found to be very effective. One of the most effective psychotherapeutic approaches for treating addiction is cognitive behavior therapy (CBT) which involves a combination of behavior modification and cognitive techniques. CBT is also effective in relapse prevention.

CBT works on the underlying assumption that learning and cognitive processes play an important role in the development and continuation of substance abuse and dependence.

These same learning processes can be used to help individuals reduce their drug use. The therapist helps patients recognize the situations in which they are most likely to use drugs, avoid these situations when appropriate, and cope more effectively with a range of problems and problematic behaviours associated with substance abuse (Carroll, 1998). CBT thus, involves functional analysis, skills training and relapse prevention. It uses a variety of techniques including

Table 8.1:The Twelve Steps of Alcoholics Anonymous

1	We admitted we were powerless over alcohol—that our lives had become unmanageable
2	Came to believe that a Power greater than ourselves could restore us to sanity.
3	Made a decision to turn our will and our lives over to the care of God as we understood Him.
4	Made a searching and fearless moral inventory of ourselves.
5	Admitted to God, to ourselves, and to another human being the exact nature of our wrongs.
6	Were entirely ready to have God remove all these defects of character.
7	Humbly asked Him to remove our shortcomings.
8	Made a list of all persons we had harmed, and became willing to make amends to all.
9	Made direct amends to such people wherever possible, except when to do so would injure them or others.
10	Continued to take personal inventory and when we were wrong promptly admitted it.
11	Sought through prayer and meditation to improve our conscious contact with God, as we understood Him, praying only for knowledge of His will for us and the power to carry that out.
12	Having had a spiritual awakening as the result of these Steps, we tried to carry this message to alcoholics, and to practice these principles in all our affairs.

Copyright: A.A. World Services, Inc.

aversion treatment, behavioural contracts, mindfulness training, modelling, relaxation training, social skills training, and stress management. Individuals keep records of their success with different strategies and modify them as and when needed. To prevent relapse, individuals are helped to identify potential high-risk situations in advance and be satisfied that they are capable of managing these situations without suffering a setback in their recovery (Carrol, 1998; Somers, 2007).

Management of co-morbidities

Co-morbidities of substance abuse can be psychiatric or physical and should be managed concurrently. Some substances of abuse can be associated with psychiatric problems. It is not uncommon to find substance abusers presenting with schizophrenia-like symptoms, bipolar affective psychosis, delirium, hallucinosis, paranoid psychosis, encephalopathies, anxiety, depressive illness, dementia, personality disorders etc. It is very necessary therefore that proper Psychiatric assessment and appropriate diagnoses are made. The treatment and management of these conditions should be in line with conventional treatment for these conditions.

Physical co-morbidities can manifest as injuries to the body, infections including HIV, electrolyte imbalance, gastro-enteritis, cardio-vascular diseases, poly-neuropathies, liver and pancreas diseases. It is also very important that physical and laboratory investigations are made during assessment. Physical co-morbidities identified should be referred for appropriate attention.

Response of Government of Ghana to drug abuse

1. Establishment of the Narcotics Control Board (NACOB) and the enactment of PNDC Law 236 in 1990 with emphasis on Enforcement, Education/ Prevention, Treatment and the establishment of Rehabilitation Committees.
    i) Enhanced International cooperation, increased recruitment and training of personnel for enforcement and Demand Reduction Programmes for NACOB.

ii) School programmes for awareness creation and inclusion of drug abuse in the curricula of the Ghana Education Service.

2. Creation of the Addictive Diseases Unit at the Korle Bu Teaching Hospital in 1991. Treatment is based on the medical model and application of Alcoholic Anonymous 12 steps. The unit is supported by the Department of Psychiatry of the Medical School.
3. Ghana's three Psychiatric Hospitals apply the medical model for treatment. Main activities involve detoxification, treatment of co-morbidities, counseling and rehabilitation.
4. Counseling through efforts of Community Psychiatric Nurses.
5. Private and community-based services: A few private clinics and NGOS are involved in demand reduction efforts. These include Valley View Clinic, Peace Be Clinic (Detoxification and Treatment), Progressive Life (Centre for Psychotherapy), Remar Centre (Rehabilitation and Religious Counseling) Hopeful Way Foundation (Halfway House) and House of St. Francis (Residential Facility) for alcohol-dependent persons incorporating the 12 steps of AA.

Way forward

Addiction is a complex disease and no one factor can predict who will become an addict. Thus prevention should be the focus. Preventive programmes must address issues holistically. For instance prevention programmes in schools should focus on children's social and academic skills, including enhancing peer relationships, self-control, coping skills, social behaviours, and drug offer refusal skills.

Other services ought to include:

a. Provision of national treatment and rehabilitation centres outside the psychiatric hospitals with trained personnel dedicated to the management of substance abusers.
b. Management of substance use disorders at primary, district regional and national levels (Mental Health Act 846, Section 1 Article 3 (d)). This would involve training more people, and

working closely with District Assemblies and others in the community in the management of drug users.

c. A national programme for the management of substance abuse under an independent commission which should be resourced using a multidisciplinary team.

References

Affiniih, Y. (1999). Drug Use in Greater Accra: A Pilot Study. *Substance Use & Misuse*, *34*(2), 157-1 69.

Asare, J.B, (1999.) Alcohol Use, Sale and Production in Ghana: A health Perspective. In: S. Peel & M. Grant (Ed.) *Alcohol for Pleasure*, p. 121-130.

Asare, J.B. (2008).*The problem of Drug abuse in Ghana* Monograph, Sedco Publishers.

Asare, J. B. (2009). *Overview of Substance Abuse in Ghana*. Available at: hopefulway.webs.com/AsareOverview20-24April.doc

Asare, J. B., & Wellington, E. (2004). Baseline Survey of Existing Relationship between HIV Infection and Substance Abuse in Ghana. UNODC Document 2004.

Atwoli. L., Mungla P., Ndung'u M., Kinoti K. & Ogot E. (2011). Prevalence of substance use among college students in Eldoret, Western Kenya. *BMC Psychiatry* 11:34. Available at: http://www.biomedcentral.com/1471-244X/11/34.

Brannon, F., & Jess, F. (2004) *Health Psychology: An Introduction to Behavior and Health* (5th Ed.). Thomson Wardsworth.

Bahr, S.J., Hoffman, J.P., & Yang, X. (2005). Parental and Peer Influences on the Risk of Adolescent Drug Use. *The Journal of Primary Prevention, 66 (2): 161-182.*

Carroll, K.M. (1998). Therapy Manuals for Addiction: A Cognitive Behavioural Approach for Treating cocaine Addiction. Available at:http://archives.drugabuse.gov/TXMmanuals/CBT/CBT1.htlm

Clarke, T.T., Belgrave, F. Z.& Abell, M.(2012). The Mediating and Moderating Effects of Parent and Peer Influences upon Drug Use among African American Adolescents. Journal of Black Psychology 38(1), 52-80

Dennis-Antwi, J., Adjei, S., Asare, J.B., & Twene, R. (2003). *A National Survey on Prevalence and Social Consequences of Substance Use among Second*

Cycle and Out Of School Youth in Ghana. Available at: www.afro.who.int/index.php?option=com_docman&task.

Doku, D., Koivusilta, L., & Rimpela, A. (2012). Socioeconomic Differences in Alcohol and Drug Use among Ghanaian Adolescents. *Addictive Behaviours, 37*, 357-360.

Government of Ghana. (2012). The Mental Health Act, 2012- Act 846.

Hammond, P. (2004) *Alcohol Abuse in South Africa*. Vol 1. Available at: http://christianaction-org-za.win07.glodns.net/firearmnews/2004-01_AlcoholAbuseinSA.htm.

Hawkins, J.D., Catano, R.F., & Miller, J.Y. (1992). Risk and Protective Factors for Alcohol and Other Drug Problems in Adolescence and Early Adulthood: Implications for Substance Abuse Prevention. *Psychological Bulletin, 112*(1), 64-105

International Narcotic Control Board (2006). The *Report of the International Narcotics Control Board for 2006* (E/INCB/2006/1). Available at:http://www.incb.org/documents/Publications/AnnualReports/AR2006AR_06_English.pdf.

Kinney, J., (2003). *Loosening the Grip: A Handbook of Alcohol Information*. (7th Ed.). McGraw Hill.

Kovacs, E., Franciska, B., & Fitzpatrick, K. M. (2011). Religiosity as a Protective Factor against Substance Use among High School Students. *Substance Use and Misuse 46*, 1346–1357.

National Institute of Drug Abuse (2003). Preventing Drug Use among Children and Adolescents: A Research-Based Guide for Parents, Educators and Community Leaders. Available at: http://www.drugabuse.gov/sites/default/files/preventingdruguse.pdf.

Pary, C.D. (1998). *Substance Abuse in South Africa: Country Report Focussing on the Youth* WHO/UNDCP. Avaiable at: http://www.sahealthinfo.org/admodule/countryreport.pdf.

Ray, O., & Ksir, C. (2004). *Drugs and Society and Human Behavior*. (10th Ed.). Boston:McGraw Hill.

Somers, J., & Queree, M., (2007). Cognitive Behavioural Therapy: Core Information Document. Available at: http://www.health.gov.bc.ca/library/publications/year/2007/MHA_CognitiveBehaviouralTherapy

The National Centre on Substance Abuse (2011). *Adolescent Substance Use: America's #1 Problem*. Available at: www.casacolumbia.org/upload/2011/20110629substanceseslides.pdf.

The Twelve Steps of Alcoholic Anonymous. (2002) http://www.aa.org/en_pdfs/smf-121_en.pdf.

UNODC (2012). *West Africa ATS Situation Report*. Available at: http/www.unodc copy of ATS West Africa final.

UNODC (2012). *World Report on Drugs*. Available at: http://www.unodc.org/documents/data-and analysis/WDR2012/WDR_2012_web_small.pdf.

Wellington, E. (2000).*Ghana Global Youth Tobacco Survey (GYTS). Available at:*http://www.afro.who.int/indexphp?option=com_docman& task=doc_download&gid=1886.

Wellington, E. (2005). *Ghana Global Youth Tobacco Survey. Available at:* www.afro.who.int/index.php?option=com_docman&task

Wellington, E. (2006). *Ghana Global Youth Tobacco Survey*. Available at: www.afro.who.int/index.php?option=com_docman&task

WHO (2000). Primary *Prevention of Substance Abuse: A Facilitator Guide,* (WHO/MSD/MDP/00.18). *Available at* http://www.who.int/substance_abuse/activities/global_initiative/en/primaryprevention-guide 17.pdf

WHO (2000). *Primary Prevention of Substance Abuse: A Workbook for Project Operators,*(WHO/MSD/MDP/00.17).Available at:http://www.who.int/substance_abuse/activities/global_initiative/en/primary_prevention_17.pdf.

WHO (2011). *WHO Status Report on Alcohol and Health 2011. Retrieved from* http://www.who.int/substance_abuse/publications/global_alcohol_report/profiles/gha.pdf.

WHO. (2012). *Management of Substance Abuse: Facts and Figures*. Available at: http://www.who.int/substance_abuse/facts/en/index.html

WHO. (2012). *HIV Fact Sheets*. Available at: http://www.who.int/mediacentre/factsheets/fs360/en/index.html

Chapter 9

Schizophrenia in Primary Care

David Goldberg, Gabriel Ivbijaro, Lucia Kolkiewicz and Sammy Ohene

Introduction

Schizophrenia is the name given to a group of mental disorders in which delusions and hallucinations predominate, and there are alterations in a person's perception, thoughts, feelings and behavior. Each person with the disorder will have a unique combination of symptoms and experiences. Typically, there is a *prodromal period*, often characterized by some deterioration in personal functioning. This period may include memory and concentration problems, unusual behavior and ideas and disturbed communication and affect. Schizophrenia affects approximately 7 per 1,000 people from adolescence onwards. It is an illness with low incidence and high prevalence, due to the effects of chronicity, and is of importance to primary care because of a shortage of mental health specialists globally, especially in low- and middle-income countries (WHO, 2005). In most countries, whatever their income, primary care will be the first contact for many people who suffer from mental health conditions (WHO & Wonca, 2008).

Historical background

Schizophrenia has been noted in all cultures throughout recorded history. In the 19th century, the French psychiatrist Benedict Morel, who observed rapid intellectual deterioration in a young teenage boy from a good student to one with confused thoughts and grossly disorganized behavior over a few months, named the disorder *démence précoce* (Morel, 1860). In 1893, the fourth edition of Emil Kraepelin's textbook *Psychiatrie* introduced *dementia praecox* under the heading of "Psychic degenerative processes" (Kraepelin, 1893).

In 1911, Eugene Bleuler replaced the term "*dementia praecox*" with "schizophrenia", because he believed the cognitive impairment associated with the disorder arose from splitting of psychic function

(Bleuler 1911). Bleuler identified in his Companion to Primary Care Mental Health; four disturbances, known as "the four As", as fundamental to the disorder. These were **A**ffective blunting, loosening of **A**ssociation, **A**utism and **A**mbivalence. He considered hallucinations and delusions as nonspecific to the diagnosis of schizophrenia, since they occurred in patients with other conditions such as manic depressive (bipolar) illness.

In 1959 Kurt Schneider, a German psychiatrist, drew attention to the importance of psychotic symptoms in the diagnosis of schizophrenia and identified certain "first-rank" psychotic symptoms as diagnostic, thus introducing greater objectivity and specificity into the diagnostic process (Schneider 1959). First-rank symptoms included thought insertion, thought withdrawal, thought broadcasting, delusions of control, audible thoughts, voices arguing about a subject, voices commenting on actions in the third person and delusional perception.

Epidemiology of schizophrenia

Schizophrenia is an illness with an unclear aetiology, which is likely to be both complex and multifactorial and to involve a gene and environment interaction. The best way to consider this in a primary care setting is by adopting a life-course approach, which begins from genetics, obstetric complications, childhood adversity, adolescent adversity and other life events of adulthood.

There is an association between schizophrenia and family history, as having a first-degree relative with schizophrenia increases a person's likelihood of experiencing schizophrenia ten-fold, while having two affected parents or an affected twin confers a likelihood of 50 percent (Kendler & Diehl, 1993). There is also evidence that prenatal infections can be associated with schizophrenia; these include rubella (Brown, Cohen & Harkvay. Friedman 2001), influenza (Brown et. al, 2004) and toxoplasmosis (Brown, Mcleod, 2005). One of the theories proposed to explain this association is the role of cytokine and chemokine as mediators of the host response to infection (Buka, Cannon& Torrey, 2001). In addition to obstetric infections, other obstetric complications may be associated with an increased incidence of schizophrenia (Crow 2003). There is evidence that childhood trauma may be associated with psychosis (Read, Van Os & Morrison, 2005). However, Morgan and Fisher (2007) are of the opinion that a number of conceptual and methodological issues need to be addressed before a definite conclusion can be reached. Adolescent and adult psychosocial stressors, including first- and second-generation migration (Cantor-Graae & Selten, 2005 ; Coid , Kirkbride& Baker, 2008) inner city environment (Van Os, Driessen & Gunther 2000; Van Os, Hanssen & Bijl, 2001 & Sundquist, 2004) and, in some cases, substance misuse (Andréasson et. al, 1987; Philips & Johnson, 2001; Batel, 2000), are all associated with onset, maintenance and relapse of schizophrenia. The incidence of schizophrenia is higher in men than in women (Castle, Wessley & Murray, 1993; Iacono & Beiser, 1992). In summary, there is a need for a bio psychosocial approach to the management of schizophrenia.

Prevention starts with:

- genetic counseling for those parents who have a high genetic risk;
- prevention of infections in the prenatal period;
- good obstetric care during delivery;
- prevention of childhood trauma and deprivation;
- support for migrants;
- good environmental planning to decrease the stress of living in inner cities.

Positive and negative symptoms

There are two main groups of symptoms, and both may be present simultaneously or each can occur on their own. The prodromal period is usually followed by an acute episode marked by *positive symptoms* such as hallucinations, delusions and behavioural disturbances, accompanied by agitation and distress. *Negative symptoms* may take the form of social withdrawal, apathy and reduced interest in daily activities. In those with prolonged illnesses, there may be some cognitive decline over many years.

Acute episodes and persistent states

The *International Classification of Diseases* (ICD)-11 for primary health care (ICD11-PHC) is due to be released by the World Health Organization (WHO) in 2014. It distinguishes between acute episodes of psychosis and persistent psychotic states, where the illness has not resolved fully and may display both positive and negative features. The concept of "acute psychosis" includes transient psychotic states that last less than one month, as well as schizophrenia, which is the name given to illnesses that have lasted more than one month. For primary care purposes, the broader concept is preferable, as an individual primary care clinician is more likely to see cases of transient psychotic states than first onset of schizophrenia. Since schizophrenia is often a long-lasting disorder, primary care clinicians are most likely to see cases of persistent psychotic illness.

Acute psychotic disorder

Presenting symptoms and complaints

Patients can present with sudden onset of severe disturbance, characterized by strange beliefs and grossly abnormal behavior. They may be apprehensive, confused or extremely suspicious. Acute psychosis can be very transient in nature, lasting for a few hours to a few days, or can last for a few weeks. Complete recovery is the norm. *Schizophrenia should not be diagnosed until the disorder is still present after 4 weeks.* It is often very difficult to know the extent to which drugs may be responsible for psychotic experiences, and patients should always be asked what drugs they have used in recent weeks.

Required symptoms:

- Delusions (strange beliefs may involve being persecuted or poisoned, of special powers, of one's spouse's infidelity, of being controlled or of being talked about by strangers);
- Hallucinations (hearing voices or seeing visions).

Other common symptoms

- Withdrawal;
- Agitation, restlessness or disorganized behavior;
- Muddled thinking;
- Incoherent or irrelevant speech;
- Labile emotional states.

Differential diagnosis

- Bipolar disorder – the manic phase and psychotic forms of depression may have many similar features; patients may develop symptoms of classical mania and depression or may go on to become chronic, mandating a change in diagnosis over time.
- Drug-induced psychotic states ;
  - Exacerbations of a persistent psychosis, with a total duration of illness of more than 3 months;
  - Medical conditions such as delirium, with systemic or cerebral infections, and epilepsy.

Persistent psychotic disorder

Presenting symptoms and complaints

The presentations include abnormal beliefs, hearing voices or seeing visions and may involve abnormal behavior. Patients can also present with lack of energy for daily chores, lack of motivation to work, difficulty in concentrating, apathy and withdrawal from family, friends and colleagues.

Diagnostic features

Acute exacerbations include:

- delusions (strange beliefs of being persecuted or poisoned, of special powers, of one's spouse's infidelity, of being controlled or of being talked about by strangers);
- hallucinations (hearing voices and seeing things that others cannot see);

- restlessness and agitation;
- grossly abnormal behaviour.

Persistent problems include:

- lack of energy or motivation to carry out daily chores and work
- apathy and social withdrawal,
- strange and abnormal speech,
- poor personal care or neglect.

Differential diagnosis

- Bipolar disorder – the manic phase may have many similar features;
- Psychosis can also be associated with medical illnesses (e.g. infections and tumors of the brain, head injury, epilepsy, thyroid disorder);
- Dementia – organic psychoses (e.g. dementia) can have similar features;
- Substance use – e.g. alcohol, cannabis, opioids, etc.

Interviewing and assessing a psychotic patient

Time is always short in primary care, and you may have to speed up your assessment. Some basic strategies to follow:

- The patient must perceive you as their own doctor, rather than the agent of their parents. If the patient is accompanied, start your interview with the patient, and only take a history from others with the patient's consent. Listen to the patient's account of the present problem, with sympathy and encouragement. If the patient is not sure why he or she has come, ask what has worried other people and suggested that they visit. If you are still not making much progress, ask whether the patient has had any experiences they could not account for, or has had any recurrent thoughts that troubled them.
- If odd experiences are described, ask if they were taking any drugs at the time, or whether they have experimented with them in the last few weeks. If you are still making little progress

and they are accompanied, ask if they mind asking the person with them what they have noticed that worries them.

- In any case, you will need to take control of the interview and do a quick ***mental state examination***. How are they feeling at present? Are they worried about themselves? Have they felt that life isn't worth living? (***If so, have they had thoughts about harming themselves?***) Have they found that they can hear things that other people don't seem to hear? Or have they seen things that they couldn't account for? (***Have they had auditory or visual hallucinations: can they describe what they have heard/seen?***) Have they had any problems with their thinking (***thoughts inserted, or controlled by others***)? Can they tell you where they are, what date/day of week it is, and who you are (***orientation***)?

Management of schizophrenia in primary care

The management of schizophrenia requires an integrated approach that recognizes the central importance of the patient, their family and care givers, is holistic, and focuses on developing patient strengths and promoting recovery. Management of schizophrenia requires recognition that the person with schizophrenia is an individual who should be treated with respect and empowered to manage the illness, so that they can maintain hope and obtain treatment in the least restrictive environment possible, and live a satisfying, hopeful and contributing life, despite the limitations caused by illness (Anthony, 1993).

As with all other mental health conditions, it is important to invest in manpower to improve patient access to treatment, so that mental and physical health needs are addressed in an integrated way that can deliver the best possible outcomes.

It is known that not all people with schizophrenia will visit primary care, as illustrated by Goldberg and Huxley (1992); therefore, a systematic approach to the management of schizophrenia that takes into account prevention, the subtype of schizophrenia and its course is necessary.

Low- and middle-income countries

In *middle-income countries* where secondary care mental health services are less well developed, general practitioners and family physicians should form an alliance with their local psychiatrist so that they can readily elicit support and advice to help them better manage early-onset cases of schizophrenia and those who have not responded to the usual treatment interventions. This approach can be better supported where locally agreed management guidelines have been jointly developed by primary care physicians and secondary care psychiatrists, as this will provide a clear guideline on when it is appropriate to ask for extra help or refer to the local mental health service. Liaison with mental health services can be further enhanced by organizing regular meetings between primary care staff and the local psychiatrist at the primary care clinic where complex cases can be brought and discussed. Many middle-income countries have a network of district general hospitals that provide a range of services. General practitioners and family physicians should negotiate admission rights for psychiatric patients requiring inpatient care, supported by clear admission guidelines and treatment protocols. In such circumstances, the role of the psychiatrist is to assist in developing evidence-based treatment protocols and guidelines, regular educational support and ongoing coaching to medical staff who are managing people with schizophrenia. In *low-income countries*, where primary care services and secondary care mental health services are poorly developed, the roles of the general practitioner or family physician are different, as, not only are they the first point of contact, they also have to take on the role of local specialist for a range of mental health disorders. In such situations, it is even more important for primary care to develop very detailed schizophrenia protocols and guidelines to follow. If there are other general practitioners or family physicians in the area, they should form an alliance of mutual support or cooperation, including co-mentoring and peer support. They should develop the role of health-care workers to support their mental health interventions, and work with local opinion leaders and advocates to address stigma and promote access. In some countries where traditional healers play a role, general practitioners and other health professionals working in primary care should work with their local health boards to generate a list of local traditional healers, so that they can provide them with mental health education and support, and their usefulness can be harnessed as part of the extended primary health-care team.

In all countries, there is a need to develop a local formulary of a range of medications that are affordable, and of proven benefit in the treatment of schizophrenia, so that access to pharmacological interventions can be guaranteed. The key to delivering good health is to keep the patient and their family or carer at the centre of the service.

Specific interventions for the treatment of schizophrenia

Once a history has been taken and a diagnosis made, an intervention plan should be developed using the following headings.

General

The person presenting with schizophrenia should be provided with a diagnosis and explanation of the disorder in a form that they can easily understand. All people with schizophrenia should be assessed for risk of harm to self and others.

The prodromal phase

In many parts of the world, specialized early-intervention services are not available, and primary care staff must use their own judgment in deciding what assistance to offer the person in a prodromal phase. If there is access to a local mental health service, it may sometimes be helpful to refer the patient, provided that he or she agrees to this. Where available, there are three components to the assistance a mental health service provides: first, early identification and therapeutic engagement of people in the prodromal phase; second, provision of specialized pharmacological and psychosocial interventions during or immediately following a first episode of psychosis; and third, education of the patient and his or her family and the wider community to reduce obstacles to early engagement in treatment.

An acute episode of psychosis

- For people with newly diagnosed schizophrenia presenting with positive symptoms, offer *oral antipsychotic medication*. Provide information and discuss with the service user the benefits and side-effect profile of any drug you intend to use, bearing in mind the relative potential of individual antipsychotic drugs to cause extrapyramidal side-effects (including akathisia), metabolic side-effects (including weight gain) and other side-effects (including unpleasant subjective experiences). In nine randomized controlled trials (RCTs) with a total of 1801 participants with first-episode or early schizophrenia (including people with a recent onset of schizophrenia and people who had never been treated with antipsychotic medication), the evidence suggested there were no clinically significant differences in efficacy between the antipsychotic drugs examined (National Collaboration Centre for Mental Health, 2010). These medications are effective in reducing all florid symptoms, and in reducing excited behavior.
- Referral to a specialized *mental health service* will depend upon local availability of such a service. Patients with grossly *disturbed behavior*, or where there is thought to be a danger to either the patient or to others, are usually referred. If possible, all first episodes of acute psychosis should be referred to the specialist service.
- If patients are to be *managed in the community*, it is advisable for them to be visited by a mental health nurse who is able to give advice and support to care givers. Interface with the local mental health service is facilitated if there is a *written care plan* that has been agreed between the two services and the service user and his or her family. Such care plans typically include details of symptoms both in relapse and admission, the usual medication and an acceptable alternative, details of any mental health nurse allocated to the case, and information on how to arrange readmission if this becomes necessary. There should be opportunities to have *case discussions* between primary care and mental health staff, especially at times of crisis.

- When the crisis of an acute episode is resolved, offer *family intervention* to all families of people with schizophrenia who live with or are in close contact with the service user. This is a specialized procedure best carried out by someone who has been trained to deliver such interventions. Family interventions aim to reduce the level of expressed emotion in the family and to decrease critical comments towards the patient, as well as to help care givers deal with problems and to improve knowledge about the illness in both the service user and his or her family. Therapists are most likely to be a mental health professional. In 32 RCTs including 2429 participants, there was robust and consistent evidence for the efficacy of family intervention (National Collaboration Centre for Mental Health, 2010). When compared with standard care family interventions have been shown to reduce the risk of relapse and to produce a lower level of active symptoms for up to 2 years after the intervention (Pilling et al., 2002; McGill et al., 1983).
- The National Institute for Health and Clinical Excellence (NICE) recommends that general practitioners and other primary health-care professionals should *monitor the physical health* of people with schizophrenia at least once a year. You should focus on cardiovascular disease risk assessment as described in the NICE guideline, *Lipid modification*, but bear in mind that people with schizophrenia are at higher risk of cardiovascular disease than the general population. A copy of the results should be sent to the care coordinator and/or psychiatrist, and put in the secondary care notes (National Institute for Health and Clinical Excellence, 2008).
- *Do not* initiate regular combined antipsychotic medication, except for short periods (for example, when changing medication).

Interventions for people with schizophrenia whose illness has not responded adequately to treatment

- First, review the diagnosis. Other possible explanations for symptoms include intoxications with drugs or alcohol and organic brain disease.
- Next, try to establish whether there has been adherence to antipsychotic medication, prescribed at an adequate dose and for the correct duration.
- Review engagement with and use of psychological treatments and ensure that these have been offered.

  If there is access to a specialist mental health service, ask for an opinion on which drug to try next. At least one of the drugs should be a non-clozapine second-generation antipsychotic.
- If trained staff is locally available to administer *cognitive-behavioral therapy adapted for schizophrenia* (CBTp), suggest this as next step. When compared with standard care, CBTp was effective in reducing both the rate of re-admissions to hospital and the duration of admissions. Negative symptoms were reduced at one-year follow-up (Tarrier et. al. 1988). Early CBT trials tended to be particularly symptom focused, helping service users develop coping strategies to manage hallucinations (Tarrier et. al. 1988). Since then, however, CBTp has evolved and now tends to be based on a manual. It should take place over a series of sessions, and establish links between the patient's thoughts, feelings or actions and their current or past level of functioning, and allow the patient to re-evaluate how their perceptions, beliefs or reasoning relate to the target symptoms.
- Offer *Clozapine* to people with schizophrenia whose illness has not responded adequately to treatment despite sequential use of adequate doses of at least two different antipsychotic drugs. In 18 RCTs including 2554 participants whose illness had not responded adequately to treatment, clozapine had the most consistent evidence for efficacy over the first-generation antipsychotics included in the trials (National Institute for

Health and Clinical Excellence, 2009). A number of patient-related factors have been reported to increase the variability of plasma clozapine concentrations, with sex, age and smoking behavior being the most important.

Patients with persistent psychotic states

Patients may reach a relatively stable state, with some residual positive symptoms in addition to some negative symptoms. Positive symptoms may reappear when the patient has experienced a stressful life event, or when they have stopped taking their medication. The advice given above will apply to management of the positive symptoms.

The use of depot medication

Consider this only where there is clear evidence that antipsychotic drugs are effective in controlling symptoms, and where there is evidence that the patient repeatedly relapses when medication is not taken, and agrees to receive depot medication.

In six RCTs, including 252 participants with schizophrenia, there was some evidence that clozapine augmentation with a second antipsychotic might improve both total and negative symptoms if administered for an adequate duration (Potter, Ko, Zhang et al., 1989).

Negative symptoms

There is no consistent evidence that one antipsychotic drug is any better at relieving negative symptoms than the others. In 10 RCTs including 1200 participants with persistent negative symptoms, there was no evidence of clinically significant differences in efficacy between any of the antipsychotic drugs examined (National Collaboration Centre for Mental Health, 2010). Careful clinical assessment is warranted to determine whether such persistent features are primary or secondary, and may identify relevant treatment targets, such as drug-induced Parkinsonism, depressive features or certain positive symptoms (National Institute for Health and Clinical Excellence, 2009). However, if clozapine is augmented with another antipsychotic drug, there is some evidence of efficacy, as discussed above. There are also social and psychological treatments that are effective to some extent. ***Arts therapies***, which allow expression of emotions, whether by drama, by pottery or by painting, have been shown to have such an effect. There is consistent evidence that arts therapies are effective in reducing negative symptoms when compared with any other control (National Institute for Health and Clinical Excellence, 2009). There is some evidence indicating that the medium-to-large effects found at the end of treatment were sustained at up to 6 months' follow-up (National Institute for Health and Clinical Excellence, 2009). CBTp may also reduce negative symptoms.

Social care and rehabilitation

A *social assessment* is necessary to ensure that an individual is obtaining whatever social benefits are available, and has somewhere to live that provides shelter from adverse weather, and adequate food. Social interventions for schizophrenia should include supported employment, including opportunities for volunteering (Becker et al., 2007), access to education and leisure activities and appropriate housing. Supported employment programs may provide assistance to people with schizophrenia who wish to return to work or gain employment. However, they should not be the only work-related activity offered when individuals are unable to work or are unsuccessful in their attempts to find employment. Patients with persistent psychotic disorders need to *structure their time* usefully, and gain help and support with regular social contacts, perhaps in a group setting.

Re-referral to the specialist mental health services

For a person with schizophrenia being cared for in primary care, consider referral to secondary care again if there is a poor response to treatment, non-adherence to medication, intolerable side-effects from medication, coexisting substance misuse, or risk to self or others.

Reducing the risk of relapse and the promotion of recovery

The NICE guidelines showed that in 17 RCTs including 3535 participants with schizophrenia, the evidence suggested that, when compared with placebo, all of the antipsychotics examined reduced the risk of relapse or overall treatment failure (National Collaboration Centre for Mental Health, 2010). Although some second-generation antipsychotic drugs show a modest benefit over haloperidol, there is insufficient evidence to choose between antipsychotics in terms of relapse prevention.

Conclusions, prognosis and future developments

It cannot be emphasized enough that the schizophrenic cluster of psychoses are by no means always chronic disorders. In the WHO 10-country study, it was found that, even in high-income countries, of those satisfying criteria for schizophrenia, about 37 percent may expect to have a remitting course and eventually to recover. In low- and middle-income countries, the outlook is much more positive, with 63 percent having such a favourable course (Jablensky, Schwarz & Tomov, 1980). This is despite the fact that in the former patients,were on antipsychotic drugs for more than 75 percent of the 2-year follow-up, while in the latter the corresponding figure was 16 percent. Primary care staff are therefore urged to take a positive, even modestly optimistic view of the prognosis, and this is especially true for transient psychotic disorders. Indicators of a poor outlook are a slow, gradual onset over months or years, a long duration of untreated psychosis, a poor premorbid adjustment, and a schizoid personality. One or more of Schneider's "first rank" symptoms (see earlier, "Historical background") mean that the patient will have a three-fold increased risk of relapse (Jablensky et al. 1980). The best predictor of relapse is failure to continue to take antipsychotic medication (Dencker Malm & Lepp, 1986), and those using cannabis are also at greatly increased risk of relapse (Linszen, Dingemans, & Lenior, 1994).

In contrast, a sudden onset, a severe precipitating life event, and a good adjustment during adolescence, being married, having close friends and avoiding street drugs all indicate a more favourable course (Strauss & Carpenter, 1974).

Future developments include a continuing tendency to avoid caring for these patients in large institutions, and instead to look after them in as normal as possible a social context. Negative symptoms accumulate in unstimulating environments, and they are strikingly less evident in those cared for in the community. It is likely that further advances will be made in identifying the genetic basis for schizophrenia, and, in particular, in our understanding of the social environments that interact with these genes.

References

Andréasson, S. et al. (1987). Cannabis and schizophrenia. A longitudinal study of Swedish conscripts. *The Lancet*, 330:1483–1486.

Anthony, W. A. (1993). Recovery from mental illness: the guiding vision of the mental health service system in the 1990s. *Psychosocial Rehabilitation Journal*, 17:169–170.

Batel, P. (2000). Addiction and schizophrenia. *European Psychiatry*, 15: 115–122.

Becker, D. et al. (2007). A long-term follow up of adults with psychiatric disabilities who receive supported employment. *Psychiatric Services*, 58:922–928.

Bleuler, E., (1911). *Dementia praecox or the group of schizophrenias* (translated by Zinkin L). New York: International Universities Press.

Brown, A. S. Schaefer, C. A., Quesenberry, C.P.,Babilas,V. P, Liu, L., Susser, E.S., (2005). Maternal exposure to toxoplasmosis and risk of schizophrenia in adult offspring. *American Journal of Psychiatry*, 167:767–773.

Brown, S., Begg M., Gravenstein, S., Schaefer C. Wyatt R., Bresnahan M., Babalus V., Susser E.(2004). Serologic evidence for prenatal influenza in the aetiology of schizophrenia. *Archives of General Psychiatry*, 61: 61(8):774-780. doi:10.1001/archpsyc.61.8.774.

Brown, S., Cohen P., Harkavy –Friedman, J., Babalus, V. (2001). Pre-natal rubella, premorbid abnormalities and adult schizophrenia. *Biological Psychiatry*, 49:473–486.

Buka, S. L., Cannon, T.D., Torrey, E.F., Yolken, R.H., et al. (2001). Maternal cytokine levels during pregnancy and adult psychosis. *Brain Behaviour and Immunity*, 15:411–420.

Buckley, P., Miller A., Olsen J., Garver, D., Miller, D., Csermanky,J., (2001). When symptoms persist: clozapine augmentation strategies. *Schizophrenia Bulletin*, 27:615–628.

Cantor-Graae, E. & Selten, J. P. (2005). Schizophrenia and migration: a meta-analysis and review. *American Journal of Psychiatry*, 162:12–24.

Castle, D. J, Wessley, S. & Murray, R. M. (1993). Sex and schizophrenia: Effects of diagnostic stringency, and associations with premorbid variables. *British Journal of Psychiatry*, 162:658–664.

Coid, J. W., Kirkbride J.B., Barker, D., Cowden, F., Stamps, R., Yang, M., Jones P.B., (2008). Raised incidence of all psychoses among migrant groups. *Archives of General Psychiatry*, 65:1250–1258.

Crow, T. (2003). Obstetric complications and schizophrenia. *American Journal of Psychiatry*, 135:1011– 012.

Dencker, S. J., Malm, U., Lepp, M. (1986). Schizophrenic relapse after drug withdrawal is predictable. *Acta Psychiatrica Scandinavica*, 73:181–185

Goldberg, D. P., Huxley, P. J. (1992). *Common mental disorders – a biosocial model*. London, Routledge.

Iacono, W. G. & Beiser, M. (1992). Are males more likely than females to develop schizophrenia? *American Journal of Psychiatry*, 149:1070–1074.

Jablensky, A., Schwarz, R., Tomov, T. (1980). WHO Collaborative Study of impairments and disability associated with schizophrenic disorders. *Acta Psychiatrica Scandinavica*, 62, (suppl 285), 62:152–163.

Kraepelin, E. (1893). *Psychiatrie*, 4th ed. Liepzig: J.A. Barth.

Linszen, D. H., Dingemans, P. M., Lenior, M. E. (1994). Cannabis abuse and the course of recent onset schizophrenic disorders. *Archives of General Psychiatry*, 51:273–279.

McGill, C.W., Falloon, I.R., Boyd, J.L., et al (1983) Family educational intervention in the treatment of schizophrenia. *Hospital and Community Psychiatry* 34:934–938.

Morel, B. A., (1860). *Traité de maladies mentales*. Paris: Victir Masson.

Morgan, C. & Fisher, H. (2007). Environmental factors in schizophrenia: childhood trauma- a critical review. *Schizophrenia Bulletin*, 33:3–10.

National Collaborating Centre for Mental Health, (2010). *Schizophrenia. The NICE guideline on core interventions in the treatment and management of schizophrenia in adults in primary and secondary care (update edition)*. London, Royal College of Psychiatrists and British Psychological Society.

National Institute for Health and Clinical Excellence, (2009). *Schizophrenia: core interventions in the treatment and management of schizophrenia in adults in primary and secondary care* (update). London, (CG82).

National Institute for Health and Clinical Excellence, 2008 (CG67).*Lipid modification: cardiovascular risk assessment and the modification of blood lipids for the primary and secondary prevention of cardiovascular disease*. London.

Phillips, P. & Johnson, S. (2001). How does drug and alcohol misuse develop among people with psychotic disorder? A literature review. *Social Psychiatry and Psychiatric Epidemiology*, 36:269–276.

Pilling, S., Bebbington, P., Kuipers, E., Garety, P., Geddes, J., Orbach, G. & Morgan, C. (2002). Psychological treatments in schizophrenia: Meta analysis of family intervention and cognitive behaviour therapy. *Psychological Medicine*, 32:763–782.

Potter, W. Z. Ko, G.N., Zhang, L.D., & Yan, W. (1989). Clozapine in China: a review and preview of US/PRC collaboration. *Psychopharmacology*, 99:S87–S91.

Read, J., Van Os, J., Morrison, A. P., Ross, C.A., (2005). Childhood trauma, psychosis, and schizophrenia: a literature review with theoretical and clinical implications. *Acta Psychiatr Scand:* 112: 330–350.2005 Blackwell Munksgaard.

Schneider, K. (1959). *Clinical psychopathology*. New York: Grune & Stratton.

Kendler, K. S. and Diehl, S. R., (1993). The genetics of schizophrenia: A current, genetic epidemiological perspective. *Schizophrenia Bulletin*, 19:261–285.

Strauss, J. S., & Carpenter, W. T. Jr. (1974). Relationships between predictor and outcome variables: a report from the WHO international pilot study of schizophrenia. *Archives of General Psychiatry*, 31:37–42.

Sundquist, K., Frank, G. and Sundquist J. (2004). Urbanisation and incidence of psychosis and depression. Follow up study of 4.4 million women and men in Sweden. *British Journal of Psychiatry*, 184:293–298.

Tarrier, N.; Barrowclough, C.; Vaughn, C.; Bamrah, J .S.; Porceddu, K.; Watts, S.; and Freeman, H.L.et al. (1988). The community management of schizophrenia: a controlled trial of a behavioural intervention with families to reduce relapse. *British Journal of Psychiatry*, 153:532–542.

Van Os, J., Hanssen M., & Bijl, R.M et al. (2001). Prevalence of psychotic disorder and community level of psychotic symptoms: an urban – rural comparison. *Archives of General Psychiatry*, 58(7):663–668.

Van Os, J., Driessen G., Gunther, N. & Delespaul, P. (2000). Neighbourhood variation sin incidence of schizophrenia. Evidence for person-environment interaction. *British Journal of Psychiatry*, 176:243–248.

World Health Organization and Wonca, 2008. *Integrating mental health into primary care. A global perspective*. Geneva, World Health Organization.

World Health Organization, 2005. *Mental health atlas*, revised edition. Geneva, World Health Organization.

Section C

Mental health practice in a teaching hospital setting

Chapter 10

Liaison Psychiatry in Korle Bu Teaching Hospital

Patrick Boateng, Angela Ofori-Atta and Sammy Ohene

Introduction

The word Liaison is a French word meaning 'bonding'. When 'liaison' is used in English it means to communicate between two groups or to cooperate or work together. According to blogger Michelle Tempest (2007), 'Liaison psychiatry is a subspecialty of Psychiatry which provides consultation for psychiatric treatment to patients attending general hospitals, dealing directly at the interface between mental and physical health'. The Royal College of Psychiatrists for the UK defines Liaison Psychiatry as the sub-specialty which provides psychiatric treatment to patients attending general hospitals, whether they attend out-patient clinics, accident & emergency departments or are admitted to in-patient wards. Therefore liaison psychiatry deals with the interface between physical and psychological health.

A liaison psychiatrist is a qualified medical doctor with expertise in diagnosis and management of:

- Psychiatric illness in a medically ill patient ;
- Psychiatric illness and other psychological factors that interfere with recovery from medical illness;
- Bodily symptoms that are not adequately explained by underlying physical illness;
- Use of psychiatric drug treatment and psychological therapies in the context of physical illness; and liaison psychiatrists treat patients who present with self-harm, with medically unexplained symptoms and physical illnesses with psychological co-morbidity (Laugharne and Flynn, 2013).

Why liaison psychiatry?

This subspecialty has emerged as a result of the increasing numbers of patients with physical illness who later develop psychological illness.

Some patients with chronic physical illness such as irritable bowel syndrome, fibromyalgia, HIV/AIDS, renal impairment, burns etc. are at increased risk of developing psychological morbidities, especially mood and anxiety disorders (Grover & Kate, 2013). Also, some patients who end up at the general hospital may have unexplained or undiagnosed somatic symptoms which often leads to their being subjected to high levels of diagnostic investigation and unnecessary and costly referrals to secondary care (Naylor & Bell, 2010). Liaison psychiatry circumvents these long journeys through the physical health care services and brings relief quickly, thus saving patients and hospitals money.

Furthermore, mental illness may mimic physical illness and vice versa. Some diseases of the skin for instance, can be purely cutaneous or psychiatric in nature and this has led to the emergence of subspecialties like psycho-dermatology (Shenoi, Prabhu, Nirmal et. al., 2013). Most patients with medically unexplained symptoms or a functional somatic syndrome tend to have higher prevalence of personality disorders than the general population and may therefore require psychiatric assessment. (Laugharne et al. 2013)

Evolution of liaison psychiatry

Liaison psychiatry has evolved from historically two separate practices where individuals with mental illness were housed in large asylums and the management of those with nervous disorders were treated by physicians and neurologists in a general hospital setting (Lloyd & Mayou, 2003). Liaison psychiatry, requires skills in the assessment and management of patients with psychiatric and physical co morbidity and with complicated functional somatic symptoms. Liaison Psychiatry provides an essential service that helps bridge the gap between the physical and mental health needs of patients and this has become necessary considering the increasing pattern of somatic and mental illness (Dorogi, Campiotti & Gebhard, 2012)

The structure of liaison psychiatry in KBTH

The team involved in liaison psychiatry at Korle Bu Teaching Hospital (KBTH) comprises psychiatrists, clinical psychologists, graduate students in clinical psychology, residents in psychiatry, medical officers, general nurses and senior house officers. All staff, except residents, graduate students, medical officers and senior house officers and nurses are hired by the Medical School.

The various departments of KBTH are provided each month with a timetable giving details about doctors who are on call each day of the week. Whenever a department in the hospital has a psychiatric emergency, the first doctor on call is the House Officer. After a thorough assessment of the case, the House Officer then discusses the case with either the Medical Officer or the Resident who then gives instructions as to the management of the patient. The Consultant is subsequently informed either immediately or later depending on the complexity of the case. The patient is then reviewed by the psychiatry team on the ward as needed. Upon discharge from the ward, the client is reviewed at the Department of Psychiatry, and the next appointment is scheduled.

Patients referred from KBTH

Below is the analysis of patients seen in the Department of Psychiatry who were referred from KBTH between 2009-2012. No data is included of patients referred from other hospitals. The data includes the referring departments, age, sex and referring diagnosis. They were obtained from records at the Department of Psychiatry. There were 180 referrals during this time period, of which 66.7 percent were women and 33 percent men.

Fig 10.1: Age distribution of in-patients referred from KBTH to the Department of Psychiatry between 2009-2012

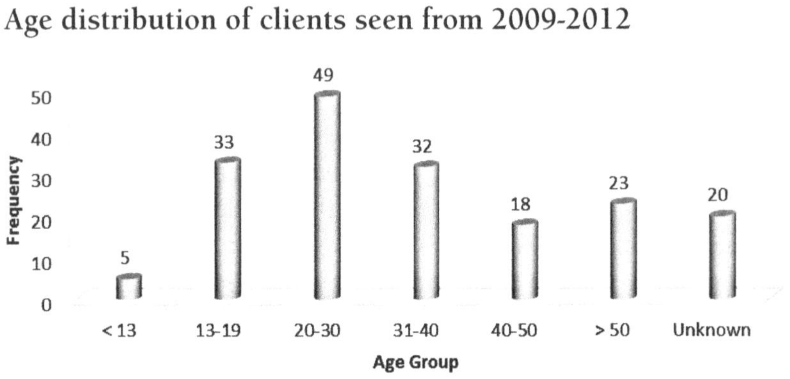

Table 10.1: Referring Departments

Department	Number of patients	Percent
Cardiothoracic Centre	1	0.6
Child Health	5	2.8
Accident and Emergency Centre	35	19.5
Ear, Nose and Throat	2	1.1
Fevers Unit	6	3.3
Genitourinary Unit	1	0.6
Gynaecology	7	3.9
Medicine	77	42.8
Neuro-Surgery	3	1.7
Obstetric	12	6.7
Orthopaedic	2	1.1
Plastic Surgery	4	2.2
Renal Unit	2	1.1
Surgical Ward	**23**	**12.8**
Total	180	100%

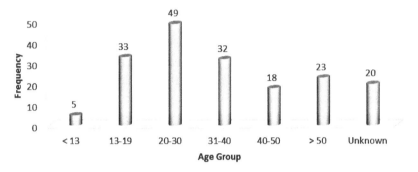

Most of the referral cases were from the departments of Medicine (42.8 percent), Accidents and Emergency (19.5 percent) and Surgery (12.8 percent). There are several reasons;department of medicine and surgery sees patients with serious chronic illness such as cancers; secondly, the emergency room is the converging point for all kinds of cases including psychiatric emergencies such as attempted suicides.

Table 10.1 shows the diagnoses given by referring doctors. The three top referring diagnoses were; **psychoses** (27%), **mood disorders** (37 %) and **anxiety disorders** (5.5 %). If it is assumed that suicidal ideation and suicidal attempts are associated with depression, then the two categories may be collapsed into one. Since suicide is a risk factor of depression, it can be assumed that depression may be responsible for 37 percent or just over one third of referrals. This is the largest single category of diagnoses and is to be expected in a Liaison Psychiatry practice; people dealing with chronic physical illness do get depressed.

The next category is Psychoses which comprises 27 percent of referred patients. This category included delusional disorder, acute psychosis, psychiatric illness, Schizophrenia and Dementia.

24 percent of patients were referred for psychological assessment or evaluation. The 5.5 percent referred for anxiety disorders included Generalized Anxiety Disorder, Panic Attacks and Phobias.

Table 10.2: Referring Diagnoses by sex from KBTH 2009-2012

Referring Diagnosis	Gender		Total
	Female	Male	
Psychotic illness	29	18	48
Suicidal thought and attempt	29	15	44
Psychological assessment	32	12	44
Mood disorders (+ 1 case of mania)	13	9	22
Anxiety disorders	5	5	10
Insomnia	1	0	1
Malingering	1	0	1
Mental Retardation	1	0	1
Post-Partum Depression	2	0	2
Rape and Sexual Abuse	2	0	2
Seizure Disorders	4	0	4
Substance Abuse	0	1	1
Torticolis	1	0	1
Total	**120**	**60**	**180**

Ways forward for liaison psychiatry in Korle Bu

The practice of liaison psychiatry in KBTH has come to stay. There is, however, the need to inform the various departments about this service to reduce the delay in referring cases.

One way to grow the subspecialty is to offer psychiatry to the College of Physicians and Surgeons as a requirement for the continuing education of physicians. This had already begun in April 2013 with topics such as ICD 10 diagnosis in psychiatry, and ethical issues in psychiatry.

The referring diagnoses to the DOP were vague in many instances, making Table 10.2 above difficult to construct. Interestingly, Table 10.2 does not carry a single diagnosis of personality disorder and yet this population of patients is thought to be more than twice as likely to have a personality disorder as the rest of the patient population

(Laugharne et al 2013). Training primary health care physicians and providing them with standardized diagnostic tools for this purpose would help physicians diagnose these disorders with accuracy and then we could begin to study the impact of personality disorders on recovery from physical disease or the added risk which personality disorders bring to physical diseases.

KBTH is dedicating a renovated ward in the old medical block to psychiatry for the purposes of setting up a brief assessment unit. This would allow the department to admit deserving cases to ensure better observation, assessment, treatment and referral to community psychiatric nurses for management closer to their homes. This would lead to a reduction of social stigma. It would also allow primarily psychiatric cases to be treated with help from other specialties of medicine.

To support liaison psychiatry in the teaching hospital setting, there is the need for the 24- hour pharmacy to be well stocked with commonly prescribed psychiatric medication. This would help reduce the present delay in acquiring anti-psychotic medication.

There are plans for KBTH to place its health educators under the Department of Psychiatry for continuing education and management. These health educators are attached to various programmes and have been trained to give information about specific illnesses, break bad news and provide support to patients in various clinics. To make this work effectively and not to shortchange patients, KBTH will need trained clinical psychologists to work alongside health educators to provide therapeutic Behavior Medicine services, and to properly supervise the health educators as they identify and refer cases which need specialist services.

Recently, the Ghana Health Service, having finalized its definition of the career paths for psychologists, has hired its first clinical psychologists and posted them to the regions. It has also sent a circular inviting various hospitals to state how many psychologists are needed in the various departments. Such hiring of psychologists into the health service is long overdue and enables liaison psychiatry to be practiced in other district and community hospitals.

Another development in this field has been the accreditation of the DOP as a site for the training of house officers in psychiatry. This has allowed an increase in the human resources available in clinical psychiatry and will boost research capacity as well.

On the whole, liaison psychiatry has become a subspecialty which is quickly growing and gaining acceptance in KBTH. Much work however remains to be done to strengthen the integration of psychiatric services within a teaching hospital setting.

Two case studies

The cases described below have been adapted to ensure patient anonymity. One describes a case of severe burns with grave family dysfunction while the second describes a case of substance-induced psychosis leading to self mutilation.

1. Case of 30 percent Total Body Surface Area (TBSA) Burns with Acute Stress Disorder

Mrs B. was a 25 year old married woman separated from her husband with whom she had had 4 young children. She was referred to the liaison psychiatry team after a fire outbreak which left her with burns on 30% of her body surface after she had rescued her children from the fire.

Her complaints were of recurrent, intrusive, distressing recollections of the event, which recollections included images, thoughts and perceptions (flashbacks). She had difficulty falling asleep and also of staying sleep, persistent intense feeling of pain, anguish, irritability and outbursts of anger.

The psycho-social issues included separation from her husband and lack of financial support as she was wholly dependent on her in-laws for support for her 4 children.

The psychiatry team focused on reconciling the patient with her family for financial and emotional support. The husband and other family members were contacted. The Department of Social Welfare was also contacted and they helped her to acquire some of the needed medication. Her psychological problems were also ameliorated through sessions of supportive psychotherapy and she was taught pain coping techniques. The relatives were educated about the supportive role which was expected of them throughout the healing process.

2. **Schizophrenia and Substance Use Disorder** A 24 year old male university student was referred to the liaison psychiatry team from the Genitourinary Department as a case of injury to self. Client was said to have severed and swallowed his penis. He had been found unconscious in a pool of his own blood in the university hostel and been rushed to the emergency room of the near- by hospital, from where he had been rushed to KBTH.

Upon interrogation, he recalled being alone in his room doing what he termed as "general sanitation" when he heard a voice which commanded him to cut his penis. This he did with a razor and later swallowed the severed stump. He woke up to find himself in a hospital bed in KBTH. He admited using heroin, cannabis (4 'rolls' a day),cigarettes(3 packets a day). He also abused alcohol (beer, spirits, bitters etc).

Mental state examination revealed a sad mood but with full affect. Speech tone was low and not spontaneous. He had thought broadcasting and thought withdrawal. He was grandiose with auditory, visual and tactile hallucinations. He also had impaired insight and was unwilling to take medication.

Treatment with antipsychotic medication improved his insight to the point where he agreed that he had a mental illness and needed treatment. The hallucinations ceased after a few weeks. The difficulty was with persuading his family to accept a report which also included the fact that he had been a multiple substance abuser. This was because of the fear on his mother's part that he would cease to be supported financially through school should his father hear about the substance use disorder. Fortunately, for him, the genitourinary team managed to reconstruct an artificial urethra through which he could urinate. He was later discharged home to be seen on an out patient basis. This case shows how important it is for patient care to have liaison psychiatric services in general hospitals.

Conclusion

Chronic medical and surgical conditions such as diabetes, heart disease, chronic obstructive pulmonary disease and cancers have significant adverse effects on a patient's quality of life. Patients with chronic medical illness have been found to be three to four times more likely to develop a psychiatric disorder than a member of the average population (NHS Confederation, 2009). Having both a psychiatric and medical illness delays recovery from both . The presence of co-morbid psychiatric disorders can lead to decreased adherence to treatment, increased health service costs and poorer outcomes (Naylor & Bell, 2010; Fear, Sheepers, Ansell et al., 2012). There is therefore the need for liaison psychiatry services to help provide comprehensive and cost effective medical services both for the patient and the country.

References

Dorogi, Y, Campiotti C, Gebhard S, (2012). Liaison Psychiatry Nurse: The Development of supervision in Somatic Medicine Encephale. 2012. 10.007. [Epub ahead of print].

Fear, C., Scheepers, M., Ansell, M., Richards R. & Winterbottom, P. (2012). "Fair Horizon's": a person-centred, non discriminatory model of mental health care delivery. *The Psychiatrist,* 36: 25-30

Grover, S. and Kate, N. (2013). Somatic Symptoms in Consultation-Liaison Psychiatry. *Int Rev Psychiatry;* 25(1):52-64. Http://Www.Nhsconfed.Org/Publications/Documents/Liaison-Psychiatry-The-Way-Ahead.Pdf

Laugharne, R. & Flynn, A. (2013). Personality disorders in consultation-liaison psychiatry. *Curr Opin Psychiatry.* 26(1):84-9.

Lloyd, G. & Mayou R. (2003). Liaison Psychiatry or Psychological Medicine, *BJP* 183:5-7.

Mental Health Network, NHS Confederation (2009). Healthy Mind, Healthy Body: How Liaison Psychiatry Services Can Transform Quality And Productivity In Acute Settings. *Briefing*, Issue 179, www.nhsconfed.org/publications.

Naylor, C. & Bell, A. (2010) Mental Health and the productivity challenge: Improving Quality And Value For Money. http://www.kingsfund.org.uk/sites/files/kf/Mental-health-productivity-Chris-Naylor-Andy-Bell-2-December-2010.pdf Retrieved September 2013.

Shenoi, S.D., Prabhu, S., Nirmal, B., & Petrolwala, S. (2013). Our Experience In A Psycho dermatology Liaison Clinic At Manipal, India, *Indian J Dermatol.* Jan; 58(1):53-5.

Tempest Michelle (2007) ; What Is Liaison Psychiatry? The Psychiatrists' Blog . Http://Drmichelletempest.Blogspot.Com/2007/01/What-Is-Liaison-Psychiatry.Html).

Chapter 11

Neuropsychological Functioning of Adult Sickle Cell Disease Patients in Ghana

M. Ampomah, C.C. Mate-Kole, A. Ofori- Atta, A. Anum, S. Ohene, I. Ekem, J.K. Acquaye,G. Ankra-Badu, F. Sey and A. Sefa-Dedeh

Background

The recent upsurge of interest in the neuropsychology of medical conditions in the Western world has contributed to the increased awareness of neuropsychology. Neuropsychology is the study of the relationship between behaviour and the activity of the brain (Elias & Saucier, 2006). The study of the neuropsychology of medical conditions came about through extensive research with both paediatric and adult patients.

In Ghana, it has become imperative to investigate the neuropsychology of medical conditions. This helps to identify the neuropsychological deficits associated with these conditions so as to make appropriate rehabilitation recommendations to improve quality of life. One such medical condition of concern to Africa is sickle cell disease (SCD) which is recognized as the most predominant haemoglobinopathy in the world (Lourerio & Rozenfeld, 2005). In Ghana, SCD is well known as "chwechweechwe" in Ga, "ahotutuo" in Twi, "nwiiwii" in Fante and "nuidudui" in Ewe (Konotey- Ahulu, 1996).

It is estimated that 2 percent of Ghanaian children born every year have SCD and about 25 percent to 30 percent of Ghanaians are carriers (Ohene-Frempong, Oduro, Tetteh et al., 2008). In 2010, 24,000 children and adults living with SCD were registered with the Sickle Cell Clinic at Korle Bu Teaching Hospital in the nation's capital (Adult Sickle Cell Clinic, Korle Bu Records, 2011).

Globally, SCD has been a major health problem. Although SCD patients are living longer due to improvements in medical care, in

Africa, which is home to millions of SCD patients, not much has been done to help adults living with SCD enjoy good quality of life. Good quality of life would be a mirage if SCD patients develop silent cerebral infarcts which is one of the disabling complications of SCD (Briscoe, 2001).

Stroke has been found to be common in adults with SCD, with an incidence among African Americans with SCD 11 times greater than in African Americans without SCD (Adams, McKie, Hsu et al., 1998). Although the effects of overt stroke and silent infarcts have been documented in both children and adults in the developed world (Kral, Brown, & Hynd, 2001), not much has been reported in Africa, especially in Ghana. Most health workers are still in a dilemma as to whether stroke really occurs in SCD patients and whether they experience neuropsychological challenges as a result of the stroke.

The literature in Africa on SCD has focused more on the medical complications associated with the disease than on examining the neuropsychological impact of SCD in children (Ogunfowora, Olanrewaju & Akenzua, 2005; Njamnshi, Mbong, Wonkam et al., 2006). The emphasis of these studies has been on children, with little emphasis on adult sickle cell patients. This is also the general trend in the Western world. To date, in Ghana, few studies have examined the psychological impact of SCD (Okraku, Ofori-Atta, Ekem, & Acquaye, 2009). However, none of the studies have examined the neuropsychology of adult SCD patients.

In this chapter, we will examine neuropsychological functioning among adult SCD patients in Ghana. We will also investigate the nature and pattern of these neuropsychological deficits.

Consequences of sickle cell haemoglobin

SCD is known to be an autosomal recessive disorder with abnormal haemoglobin leading to chronic haemolytic anaemia with numerous clinical consequences (Jaffer, Amrallah, Ali et al., 2009). Individuals with SCD inherit abnormal haemoglobin from both parents (Konotey-Ahulu, 1996). Accordingly, studies have shown that SCD is characterized by haemolytic anaemia which traps abnormal red blood cells in the blood vessels (Dauphin-McKenzie, Gilles, Jacques, & Harrington,

2006). These result in complications such as pain episodes, cerebral infarct, strokes, organ failure, gallstones, jaundice, and leg ulcers because of oxygen-deficient blood (Kral, Brown & Hynd, 2001).

Vaso-occlusion, which is also a complication of SCD, not only results in recurrent painful episodes, but also a variety of serious organ system complications that can lead to life-long disabilities and early death. The pain episodes which occur vary in intensity, location, quality and temporal patterns and are classified as acute or chronic (Franck, Treadwell, Jacob & Vichinshy, 2002). The most common triggers for vaso-occlusive events are dehydration, infection, extreme temperature and emotional stress. Other complications include acute chest syndrome and spleen sequestration (Konotey Ahulu, 1996).

SCD adult patients not only experience physiological and neuropsychological problems but also face numerous psychosocial challenges (Schatz & Puffer, 2006). The fact that SCD is a haematological disease and is present from birth, naturally poses psychosocial challenges to those living with it (Thomas & Taylor, 2002). The various symptoms and physical deformities such as frontal bossing, protruding abdomen and thin extremities which are a peculiarity of SCD patients, increase the societal stigma. The stigma of being labelled a 'sickler' and the fear of dying, the difficulties of getting pregnant, maintaining the pregnancy and increased abortion rate all contribute to difficulty in getting marital partners and also maintaining marriages especially among women with SCD (Kabiti, 2008). Also, priapism, or prolonged painful erections leads to erectile and impotence problems in males and contribute to challenges in marriage.

Other psychological problems include somatisation, depression, anxiety and hostility (Anie, Egunjobi & Akinyanju, 2010). These psychological and psychosocial difficulties impact negatively on the quality of life of patients (Anie, 2005).

SCD, stroke and neuropsychological deficits

Neuropsychological functioning refers to cognitive abilities such as intelligence, language, memory, attention/executive functioning and visuospatial skills. Neuropsychological deficits that SCD patients present may be due to many possible mechanisms such as chronic haemolytic anaemia, strokes and poor nutrition (Brown, Buchanan, Doepke et al., 1993). Recently, extensive research has established that SCD puts the surviving patient at a higher risk of ischemic stroke, primary hemorrhagic stroke and cerebral infarctions (Ohene-Frimpong et al., 1998). However, the first to associate and describe stroke in SCD more than a century ago was Sydentricker in a 3-year-old sickle cell anaemia child (Sydentricker, Mulherin & Houseal, 1923). Yet the pathophysiology of stroke in SCD patients was first reported in 1971 by Stockman, who attributed it to the occlusion of the distal internal carotid artery (Wang, 2007). Since its discovery, more studies have implicated stroke with SCD in the Western world (Earley, Kittner, Feeser et al., 1998) and in Africa (Makani, William & Marsh, 2007), of which frontal brain damage has been more commonly implicated (Brown, Davis, Lambert et al., 2000). Increased red cell adhesions, oxidative injury of the vessel wall, and chronic and acute anaemia have been identified as the causes of stroke in SCD (DeBaun, Derdeyn, McKinstry, 2006).

Strokes in SCD patients have been identified as overt and silent cerebral infarcts (Ohene-Frempong et al., 1998; Earley et al., 1998). Overt strokes present with motor deficits, however silent infarcts occur without motor deficits. They are usually diagnosed by neuroimaging techniques and neuropsychological assessments. Although studies have reported overt stroke and its sequel neuropsychological deficits to be more severe than those deficits associated with silent infarcts (Brown et al., 2000), arguably silent infarct becomes an important issue because as many as 11 percent to 17 percent of SCD patients who are otherwise asymptomatic have silent cerebral infarcts, in the absence of any motor deficits but presenting with gross cognitive deficits (Glauser et al., 1995; Moser, Miller, Bello, et al., 1996).

A majority of studies have reported neuropsychological deficits in SCD patients to be result of stroke complication (Goonan, Goonan, Brown, Buchanan & Eckman, 1994) while other studies have reported neuropsychological deficits in SCD patients with no evidence of overt stroke (e.g. Wasserman, Wilimas, Fairclough et al. 1991). With the help of neuroimaging and neurocognitive studies (Adams, 2007), these inconsistencies have been attributed to an unrecognized brain injury and cerebral infarcts according to Armstrong, Thompson, Wang et al., (1996) and Marouf, Gupta, Haider, & Adekile (2003).

The pathophysiology of SCD, particularly in relation to the brain is known to be related to the activities of the frontal regions of the brain. It is therefore not surprising that the most common neuropsychological deficits associated with SCD include problems with attention and concentration, executive skills, verbal ability and academic challenges (Brown et al., 1993), mathematics and reading achievement difficulties (Kral et al., 2001; Nabors & Freymouth, 2002). Frontal brain infarcts in SCD have been linked to patients experiencing difficulties in rehearsal and retrieval of verbal information in working memory, and recall trials (Brandling-Bennett, White, Armstrong et al., 2003; Brown et al., 2000).

Mechanism of SCD and neuropsychological deficits

The inherited abnormal haemoglobin can cause many complications and this is as a result of the inability of the sickled erythrocytes to squeeze through the small blood vessels (Bunn, 1997). The sickled cells accumulate in the vessels and cause blockage, which deprive organs and tissues of the body of oxygen (Noll, Stith, Gartstein et al., 2001). The brain thrives on oxygen transported by blood hence the deprivation of oxygen to brain cells result in a host of neuropsychological deficits according to where the lesion occurred.

Several theories have tried to explan the causes of neuropsychological deficits among SCD patients. Among those theories are Luria's theory (Luria, 1966) and the frontal lobe hypothesis (Stuss, 2011).

Luria's theory and frontal lobe deficit hypothesis

Luria (1966, 1973) described the human brain to consist of three basic functional units that are interconnected. Due to the rich interconnections of the brain, damage to one area leads to widespread consequences because of its complex and integrated nature (Stuss, 1992). For instance, damage to the frontal lobe can disrupt normal brain activity in the other brain regions. Similarly, damage to any other region of the brain can also affect the frontal lobe. Recent neuroimaging studies have implicated frontal lobe damage in SCD (Brandling-Bennett, et al., 2003; Vichinsky, Neumayr, Gold et al., 2010). This invariably means that the frontal lobe is the area most likely to get damaged in SCD patients. Although studies like Sergeant (1992) have alluded to this, there is still insufficient evidence to support this claim since others like Kotb, Tantawi, Elsayed et al. (2006) reported the fronto-parietal temporal region to be the most affected brain areas in SCD patients. This invariably suggests that SCD patients with frontal infarcts are more likely to present with frontal lobe deficits and also deficits of the other brain areas such as memory, visuospatial challenges etc. due to the rich interconnections of the brain (Brandling-Bennett, et al. 2003; Vichinsky et al., 2010).

Another prominent theory that explains executive function deficits in SCD patients is the frontal lobe hypothesis (Stuss, 2011). Stuss reported frontal lobe damage of the brain and elucidated three frontal subcircuits. The dorsolateral frontal cortex he identified as being linked to executive functions which included verbal fluency, cognitive flexibility, response inhibition, working memory, reasoning, problem-solving, and abstract thinking (Stuss, 2011). The ventromedial circuit was reported to be responsible for motivation and damage to this region results in apathy, decreased social interaction, and psycho-motor retardation (Stuss & Levine, 2002). The orbitofrontal cortex was reported to be associated with socially appropriate behavior. In this respect, he suggested that lesions in the orbitofrontal region can cause disinhibition, impulsivity, and antisocial behavior (Cummings, 1993).

Stuss (2011) again expanded the frontal lobe theory by adding the supervisory attention model which emphasizes the role of four frontal categories (energization; executive (monitoring and task setting); emotion/behavioural regulation; and metacognition) and their corresponding behaviours following frontal lobe injuries. According to Stuss (2011), patients with superior medial damage exhibit significant deficits on speeded tasks such as difficulties with letter fluency tasks during the last 45s as compared with first 15s. He attributed these challenges to a failure of "energization", which is the process of initiation and sustaining any response (Stuss, 2011).

Similarly, he explained executive function as being characterized by monitoring and task setting processes. He reported that patients who suffered frontal lobe damage encounter difficulties in keeping track of the count of stimuli under speeded conditions. He referred to these challenges a result of poor monitoring. This model explains why SCD patients with frontal lobe damage have difficulties with letter fluency, attention tasks and word list learning tasks (Vichinsky et al., 2010; Hijmans et al., 2011).

This theory is important because in patients with SCD there is possible insult to these areas and therefore we can expect that these behaviours will be compromised. In this regard, a number of studies have been conducted to investigate the neuropsychological correlates of SCD particularly among children. In the next sections, we will review some of these studies, focusing on intellectual ability, attention and executive function, memory, language and visuospatial skills.

Neuropsychological Studies of SCD children in non-African population

A majority of studies have reported the association of neuropsychological challenges with cerebral vascular damage in children living with SCD, with less focus on the adult SCD population.

A study by Hijmans, Fijnvandraat, Grootenhuis, Geloven, Heijboer et al. (2011) examined the neuropsychological deficits in children with SCD in Amsterdam. They reported that the SCD group had lower IQ scores and showed deficits in visuo-motor functioning, visuo-spatial working memory, sustained attention and planning compared to controls.

When the relationship between illness severity, psychosocial factors and neuropsychological functioning in very young SCD children was investigated at St. Christopher's Hospital for Children in Philadelphia, it was reported that participants performed significantly lower on the neuropsychological domains as compared to the normative sample. Participants reported higher scores on memory/attention tasks than the other domains (Tarazi, 2004).

A follow-up study was conducted to investigate the neuropsychological functioning in very young SCD children in relation to psychosocial factors (Anderson, 2005). It was reported that subjects performed poorly on all neuropsychological measures as compared to published normative data. Among the psychosocial factors measured, income/education significantly correlated with neuropsychological domains however disease severity was predictive of memory and attention domain. Although neuropsychological deficits have been found in adult SCD patients, the majority of studies have focused more on children.

Neuropsychological Studies of SCD Adult patients in non-African population

Although stroke has been associated with SCD, few studies have emphasised the impact of stroke in adult SCD patients. Sano, Haggerty, Kugler et al. (1996) investigated the neuropsychological functioning in adult SCD patients with no history of stroke. The authors reported that the SCD adult group demonstrated poorer performance on timed tests of attention and construction. They also reported that individuals without MR imaging or cerebral blood flow abnormalities had cognitive deficits, suggesting that subtle neuropsychological deficits can be associated with SCD in the absence of stroke.

In a similar study Vichinsky, Neumayr, Gold et al. (2010) investigated the neurocognitive dysfunction in neurologically intact adults. The authors reported mean nonverbal function to be significantly lower in SCD patients than controls. They also reported significant differences in measures such as global cognitive function, working memory, processing speed, and executive function.

Feliu, Crawford, Edwards et al. (2011) investigated the perceptions and complaints of self-reported memory and chronic pain among adult SCD patients. They reported no significant difference in memory between males or females. However, men reported more memory challenges now than when they were younger. They also reported the association between memory and average pain intensity.

All the reviewed studies above were conducted outside Africa. In the next section we will review a few studies done in Africa examining the same issues.

Neuropsychological studies of SCD children in Africa

Ogunfowora, Olanrewaju and Akenzua (2005) investigated academic performance of children with SCD in Nigeria. The authors reported that school absences among SCD patients were significantly higher than those of siblings, yet no significant correlation was found between school absence and academic achievement of the SCD children. They however reported underachievement of SCD children and suggested that it could not be attributed to absenteeism. The authors speculated that the underachievement could be attributed to brain damage which they suggested needed further studies.

A similar study was conducted in Cameroun by Njamnshi, Mbong, Wonkam et al. (2006). They examined the contribution of neuropsychological testing to the detection and prevention of stroke in SCD Cameroonian children. The authors reported that SCD children showed mild to severe cognitive deficits in attention and working memory. They also found that in relation to age, SCD children aged 17 to 20 showed greater cognitive deficits when compared to the other age groups. They suggested that cognitive deficits increase with age.

The majority of studies in Africa have focused on children, with very few focusing on the adult population. The consequence is that the long-term neuropsychological effects of SCD are not known.

The Neuropsychological deficits among adult SCD patients in Ghana

Much of the literature on SCD in Ghana is focused on addressing the stress and coping associated with SCD (Okraku et al., 2008). There is only one study that specifically examined the neuropsychological effect of SCD among adult patients in Ghana (Ampomah, 2012). This research aimed at identifying the nature of neuropsychological deficits among adult SCD patients in Ghana. The participants for the study were recruited from the Adult Sickle Cell Clinic at Korle Bu, Accra. A large cohort (127) participants was recruited for the study; 63 adult SCD patients (34 females and 29 males) and 67 adult healthy controls (28 females and 36 males). The study comprised two groups; adult SCD group and adult healthy control group.

Various neuropsychological tests were administered to participants to assess intelligence, executive functioning, memory, language, visuospatial skills. The overall results showed that adult SCD patients obtained significantly lower scores on neuropsychological tests than the healthy controls.

For instance, adult SCD patients performed poorly on intelligence measures such as the picture completion, block design and digit symbol subtests of the Wechsler Adult Intelligence Test, the National Adult Reading Test and the reading and numerical subtests of the Wide Range Achievement Test.

Similarly, on memory tests the adult SCD patients scored lower than their healthy adult controls. For example they performed poorly on memory tests such as Recognition Memory for Words, Rey Immediate Recall subtest of the Rey Complex Figure copy test, Digit Symbol Delay subtest of the Wechsler Adult Intelligence Test and the Verbal Selective Reminding Test.

Again, the SCD patients performed poorly on executive functioning measures such as the Trail Making Test and the Modified Card Sorting Test than the adult healthy controls.

Also, the SCD patients had lower scores on the Digit Symbol and Block Design subtests of the Wechsler Adult Intelligence Test and the Rey Complex Figure copy test which taps visuospatial abilities.

Finally, the healthy controls performed better on language tests such as Boston Naming Test, COWAT and the Naming Category Test than the adult SCD patients.

Intellectual functioning of adult SCD patients in Ghana

In Ghana, adult SCD patients were reported to have intelligence deficits and also performed poorly on academic achievement tests (Ampomah, 2012). Majority of studies that link SCD to intelligence in the North American and Europe reported a decline in intelligence in children and adults (Hijman et al., 2011; Tarazi, 2004; Sano et al., 1996; Vichinsky et al., 2010) which resulted in poorer performance of SCD patients on intelligence tests than their non-SCD comparison group. Also studies such as Gold, Johnson, Treadwell, et al. (2008) and Ogunfowora et al. (2005) reported that SCD patients with intelligence deficits also perform poorly on academic achievement tests.

Intelligence deficit is expected in SCD patients but the attributable factors are usually arguable. Studies such as Hijman et al. (2011) and Vichinsky et al. (2010) have implicated the brain and other causal factors have been attributed to factors such as school absenteeism as a result of painful crisis and age (Eaton & Hofrichter, 1995; Wassermann et al., 1991). Although damage to the brain and persistent school absenteeism have been found to cause intelligence deficits, some other possible causes are socioeconomic status, maternal intelligence, poverty and family stress (Tarazi, 2004). This notwithstanding, brain damage as a result of silent cerebral infarcts cannot be ignored.

Memory abilities among adult SCD patients in Ghana

In Ghana, adult SCD patients were reported to have memory deficits in comparison to the adult healthy controls (Ampomah, 2012). Njamnshi et al. (2006) and Vichinsky et al. (2010) attributed the low memory performance of SCD patients to brain damage whiles others like Tarazi (2004) attributed it to some psychological factors such as anxiety and depression, age and SES among others.

Attention/executive functioning tests among adult SCD patients in Ghana

In Ghana, Ampomah (2012) reported significant differences in scores of SCD adult patients and adult healthy controls on executive functioning tests. The adult SCD patients performed poorly on the Trail Making Test and Modified Card Sorting Test than the comparison group. The majority of studies have reported the healthy control group to have performed better on attention and executive functioning tests than the adult SCD group (Vichinsky et al., 2010) and children's studies (Kral & Brown, 2004). Neuropsychological deficits in attention and executive functions may suggest the presence and severity of cerebral damage which is more related to the frontal lobe. These deficits may lead to inhibition, sequential processing, response monitoring and mental flexibility. Other possible factors that may affect performance on these tests are age, education, speed, visual search etc.

Visuospatial abilities among adult SCD patients in Ghana

In Ghana, significant difference in scores existed between adult SCD patients and adult non-SCD patients on tests of visuospatial abilities (Ampomah, 2012). The adult SCD patients performed poorly on Digit Symbol and Block Design subtests of the Wechsler Adult Intelligence Test and the Rey Complex Figure Copy Test. More studies on visuospatial abilities in SCD patients are characterized by mixed results. While some studies reported the existence of visuospatial deficits in adults (Sano et al., 1996) and children (Hijmans et al., 2011; Tarazi, 2004), other studies did not find any significant differences (Swift, Cohen, Hynd et al., 1989). Those who reported visuospatial deficits in SCD, for example Schatz, Brown, Pascual et al. (2001), attributed them to parietal lesions. These parietal legions were speculated to be a result of the chronicity of SCD. Subsequently, Wilde, Strauss and Tulsky (2004) reported poor performance on the Block Design subtest to be caused by lesions involving the parietal regions. Parietal lobe lesions which are responsible for visuospatial skills may have contributed to the poor performance of the adult SCD patients on visuospatial tests. Other possible factors which can be attributed to the poor performance on visuospatial tests are age, poor attention and eye problems.

Language abilities among adult SCD patients in Ghana

In the Ghanaian population adult SCD patients were reported to have performed poorly on language tests such as the Boston Naming Test, COWAT and the Naming Category Test (Ampomah, 2012). Also, comparing both groups on language tests, the majority of studies done outside Africa have reported significant differences in scores. Their findings showed that the control group performed better than the SCD group on language tests in both children (Tarazi, 2004) and adult studies (Sano et al., 1996; Vichinsky et al., 2010). Vichinsky et al. (2010) attributed the cause of the language deficits to brain damage. The educational level can also impact on performance of these tests.

In summary, adult SCD patients present with neuropsychological deficits. These neuropsychological deficits include intelligence, language, memory, executive functioning tests and visuo-spatial skills.

Implications for clinical practice

The findings have implications for clinical practice as early identification, assessment and remedial programs will help provide avenues for enhancing the quality of life of adults living with medical conditions such as SCD.

For clinical practice, it is important that neuropsychological assessment becomes part of the intervention protocol for SCD patients. This will go a long way towards identifying neuropsychological deficits early for them to be appropriately rehabilitated to maximize the ability of patients to function.

The fact that most people living with medical conditions such as SCD present with neuropsychological challenges calls for a multidisciplinary team, including a clinical psychologist and a neuropsychologist to assess, diagnose and intervene to improve the quality of life of these adult patients. This would require clinical psychologists and neuropsychologists to be employed in the sickle cell clinics that would be established in district hospitals.

References

Adams, R. J. (2007). Big strokes in small persons. *Arch Neurol.*, 64(11), 1567–1574.

Adams, R. J., McKie., V. C., Hsu, L., Files, B., Vichinsky, E., Pegelow, C., Abboud, M., Gallagher, D., Kutlar, A., Nichols, F. T., Bonds, D. R., & Brambilla, D. (1998). Prevention of a first stroke by transfusions in children with sickle cell anemia and abnormal results on transcranial Doppler ultrasonography. *New England Journal of Medicine,* 339(1), 5-11.

Adult Sickle Cell Clinic, Korle-Bu Teaching Hospital (2011, June). Sickle Cell Clinic Records.

Ampomah, M. A. (2012). *Neuropsychological Functioning among Adult Sickle Cell Patients in Ghana.* An unpublished MPhil Thesis submitted to the Department of Psychology of the University of Ghana, Legon.

Anderson, E. L. (2005). *A Prospective Examination of Neuropsychological Functioning in Preschool-Age Children with Sickle Cell Disease and its Association with Psychosocial Factors.* A Thesis submitted to the Faculty of Drexel University.

Anie, A. K. (2005). Psychological complications in sickle cell disease. *British Journal of Haematology*, 129, 723–729.

Anie, A. K., Egunjobi, E. F., & Akinyanju, O. O. (2010). Psychosocial impact of sickle cell disorder: Perspectives from a Nigerian setting. *Globalization and Health*, 6, 2.

Armstrong, F. D., Thompson, R. J., Wang, W., Zimmerman, R., Pegelow, C. H., Miller, S., Moser, F., Bellow, J., Hurtig, A., & Vass, K. (1996). Cognitive functioning and brain magnetic resonance imaging in children with sickle cell disease. *Paediatrics,* 96, 864-870.

Bernaudin, F., Verlhac, .S., Fréard, F., Roudot-Thoraval, F., Benkerrou, M., Thuret, I., Mardini, R., Vannier, J. P., Ploix, E., Romero, M., Cassé-Perrot, C., Helly, M., Gillard, E., Sebag, G., Kchouk, H., Pracros, J. P., Finck, B., Dacher, J. N., Ickowicz, V., Raybaud, C., Poncet, M., Lesprit, E., Reinert, P. H., & Brugières, P. (2000). Multicenter prospective study of children with sickle cell disease: radiographic and psychometric correlation. *Journal of Child Neurology,* 15(5), 333-343.

Brandling-Bennett, E. M., White, D. A., Armstrong, M. M., Christ, S. E., & DeBaun, M. R. (2003). Patterns of verbal long-term and working memory performance reveal deficits in strategic processing in children with frontal infarcts related to sickle cell disease. *Developmental Neuropsychology*, 24, 423–434.

Briscoe, G. (2001). The cognitive and neuropsychological impact of sickle cell anaemia: a review and update. *Journal of Psychological Practice.* 7, 88–102.

Brown, R. T., Buchanan, I., Doepke, K., Eckman, J. R., Baldwin, K., Goonan, B., & Schoenherr, S. (1993). Cognitive and academic functioning in children with sickle-cell disease. *Journal of Clinical Child Psychology*, 22, 207-218.

Brown, R. T., Davis, P. C., Lambert, R., Hsu, L., Hopkins, K., & Eckman, J. (2000). Neurocognitive functioning and magnetic resonance imaging in children with sickle cell disease. *Journal of Paediatric Psychology*, 25(7), 503-513.

Bunn, H. F. (1997). Pathogenesis and treatment of sickle cell disease. *The New England Journal of Medicine*, 337(11), 762-71.

Cummings, J. (1993). Frontal-subcortical circuits and human behavior. *Archives of Neurol.* 50, 873–880.

Dauphin-McKenzie, N., Gilles, J. M., Jacques, E., & Harrington, T. (2006). Sickle cell anaemia in the female patient. *Obstetrical and Gynaecological Survey*, 61(5), 343-52.

DeBaun, M. R., Derdeyn, C. P., & McKinstry, R. C. (2006). Aetiology of strokes in children with sickle cell anaemia. *Ment Retard Dev Disabil Res Rev.*, 12, 192–199.

Earley, C. J., Kittner, S. J., Feeser, B. R., Gardner, J., Epstein, A., Wozniak, M. A., Wityk,R., Stern, B. J., Price, T. R., Macko, R. F., Johnson, C., Sloan, M. A., & Buchholz, D. (1998). *Stroke in children and sickle-cell disease.* Baltimore: Department of Neurology, Johns Hopkins University School of Medicine.

Eaton, W. A., & Hofrichter, J. (1987). Haemoglobin S gelation and sickle cell disease. *Blood*, 70, 1245-1266.

Elias, L. J. & Saucier, D. M. (2006). *Neuropsychology: Clinical and Experimental Foundations*. Boston: Allyn Bacon.

Feliu, M. H., Crawford, R. D., Edwards, L., Wellington, C., Wood, M., Whitfield, K. E., & Edwards, C. L. (2011). Neurocognitive Testing and Functioning in Adult Sickle Cell Disease. *Haemoglobin*, 35(5–6), 476–484.

Franck, L.S., Treadwell, M., Jacob, E., & Vichinshy, E. (2002). Assessment of sickle cell pain in children and young adults using the adolescent paediatric pain tool. *Journal of Pain and Symptom Management*, 23(2), 114–120.

Glauser, T.A., Siegel, M. J., Lee, B. C., & DeBaun, M. R. (1995). Accuracy of neurologic examination and history in detecting evidence of MRI-diagnosed cerebral infarctions in children with sickle cell hemoglobinopathy. *Journal of Child Neurology*, 10, 88-92.

Gold, J. I., Johnson, C. B., Treadwell, M. J., Hans, N., & Vichinsky, E. (2008). Detection and Assessment of Stroke in Patients with Sickle Cell

Disease: Neuropsychological Functioning and Magnetic Resonance Imaging. *Paediatric Haematology and Oncology*, 25, 409–421.

Goonan, B. T., Goonan, L. J., Brown, R. T., Buchanan, I., & Eckman, J. R. (1994). Sustained attention and inhibitory control in children with sickle cell syndrome. *Archives of Clinical Neurology,* 9, 89-104.

Hijmans, C. T., Fijnvandraat, K., Grootenhuis, M. A., Geloven, N., Heijboer, H., Peters, M., & Oosterlaan, J. (2011). Neurocognitive Deficits in Children with Sickle Cell Disease: A Comprehensive Profile. *Paediatric Blood Cancer*, 56, 783–788.

Jaffer, D. E., Amrallah, F. K., Ali, K. M., Mohammed, N. A., Hasan, R. A., & Humood, Z. M. (2009). Adult sickle cell disease patients' knowledge and attitude toward the preventive measures of sickle cell disease crisis *International Journal of Nursing and Midwifery,* 1(2), 10-18.

Kabiti, I. A. (2008). Anthropometric Profiles of Homozygous Sickle Cell Children in North–Western Nigeria. *AJOL*, 11, 2.

Konotey-Ahulu, F.I.D.(1996). *The Sickle Cell Disease Patient*. Watford : Tetteh –Adomeno Company.

Kotb, M. M., Tantawi, W. H., Elsayed, A. A., Damanhouri, G. A., & Malibary, H. M. (2006). Brain MRI and CT findings in sickle cell disease patients from Western Saudi Arabia. *Neurosciences,* 11, 1, 28-36.

Kral, M. C., & Brown, R. T. (2004). Transcranial Doppler Ultrasonography and Executive Dysfunction in Children with Sickle Cell Disease. *Journal of Paediatric Psychology*, 29(3), 185–195.

Kral, M. C., Brown, R. T., & Hynd, G. W. (2001). Neuropsychological aspects of pediatric sickle cell disease. *Neuropsychology Review*, 11, 179–196.

Loureiro, M. M., & Rozenfeld, S. (2005). Epidemiology of sickle cell disease hospital admissions in Brazil. *Rev Saúde Pública.*, 39, 943-949.

Luria, A. R. (1966). *Higher cortical functions in man.* New York: Basic Books.

Luria, A. R. (1973). *The working brain.* London: Penguin.

Makani, J., Williams, T. N., & Marsh, K. (2007). Sickle cell disease in Africa: burden and research priorities. *Annals of Tropical Medicine and Parasitology*, 101(1), 3-14.

Marouf, R., Gupta, R., Haider, M. Z., & Adekile, A. D. (2003). Silent Brain Infarcts in Adult Kuwaiti Sickle Cell Disease Patients. *American Journal of Haematology*, 73, 240–243.

Moser, F. G., Miller, S. T., Bello, J. A., Peglow, C. H., Zimmerman, R. A., Wang, W. C., Ohene-Frempong, K., Schwartz, A., Vichinsky, E. P., Gallagher, D., & Kinney, T. R. (1996). The spectrum of central nervous system abnormalities in sickle-cell disease as defined by magnetic resonance imaging: A report from the cooperative study of sickle cell disease. *American Journal of Neuroradiology,* 17, 965-972.

Nabors, N. A., & Freymuth, A. K. (2005). Attention deficits in children with sickle cell disease. *Percept Mot Skills*, 95(1), 57-67.

Njamnshi, A. K., Mbong, E. N., Wonkam, A., Ongolo-Zogo, P., Djientcheu, V. D., Sunjoh, F. L., Wiysonge, C. S., Sztajzel, R., Mbanya, D., Blackett, K. N., Dongmo, L., Muna, W. F. (2006). The epidemiology of stroke in sickle cell patients in Yaounde, Cameroun. *J Neurol Sci*. 250(1–2), 79-84

Noll, R. B., Stith, L., Gartstein, M. A., Ris, M. D., Grueneich, R., Vannatta, K., & Kalinyak, K. (2001). Neuropsychological functioning of youths with sickle cell disease: comparison with non chronically ill peers *Journal of paediatric psychology*, 26(2), 69-78.

Ogunfowora, O. B., Olanrewaju, D. M., Akenzua, G. I. (2005). A Comparative Study of Academic Achievement of Children with Sickle Cell Anaemia and Their Healthy Siblings. *Journal of National Medical Association*, 97, 405-408.

Ohene-Frempong, K., Oduro, J., Tetteh, H., Nkrumah, F. (2008). Screening newborns for sickle cell disease in Ghana. *Paediatrics*, 121(Suppl 2), S120-S121.

Ohene-Frempong, K., Weiner, S. J., Sleeper, L. A., Miller, S. T., Embury, S., Moohr, J. W., Wethers, D. L., Pegelow, C. H., & Gill, F. M. (1998). Cerebrovascular accidents in sickle cell disease: rates and risk factors. *Blood,* 91, 288–294.

Okraku, O., Ofori-Atta, A., Ekem, I., & Acquaye, J. K. (2009). The effects of knowledge and health beliefs on coping amongst adult Sickle Cell Patients. *Ghana International Journal of Mental Health*, 87-105.

Sano, M., Haggerty, R., Kugler, S., Martin, B. R. N. C., Prohovnik, I., Hurlet-Jensen, A., Piomelli, S., & DeVivo, D. (1996). Neuropsychological Consequences of Sickle Cell Disease. *Neuropsychiatry, Neuropsychology, & Behavioural Neurology*, 9(4), 242-247.

Schatz, J., Brown, R. T., Pascual, J. M., Hsu, L., & DeBaun, M. R. (2001). Poor school andcognitive functioning with silent cerebral infarcts and sickle cell disease. *Neurology, 56,*1109-1111.

Schatz, J. C., & Puffer, E. (2006). Neuropsychological aspects of sickle cell disease. In R. T. Brown (Ed.), *Comprehensive handbook of childhood cancer and sickle cell disease* (pp. 449–470). New York: Oxford.

Sergeant, G. R. (1992). Sickle Cell Disease. New York: Oxford University Press.

Stuss, D. T. (1992). Biological and psychological development of executive functions. *Brain and Cognition*, 20, 8-23.

Stuss, D. T. (2011). Functions of the frontal lobe: relation to executive functions. *Journal of International Neuropsychological Society,* 17, 759-765.

Stuss, D. T., & Levine, B. (2002). Adult clinical neuropsychology: Lessons from Studies of the Frontal Lobes. *Annu. Rev. Psychol.*, 53, 401–33

Swift, A. V., Cohen, M. J., Hynd, G. W., Wisenbaker, J. M., McKie, K. M., Makari, G., & McKie, V. C. (1989). Neuropsychologic impairment in children with sickle cell anaemia. *Paediatrics*, 84(6), 1077-1085.

Sydenstricker, V. P., Mulherin, W. A., & Houseal, R. W. (1923). Sickle cell anaemia. *American Journal of Diseases of Children,* 26, 132–154.

Tarazi, R. A. (2004). *Neuropsychological functioning in preschool-aged children with sickle cell disease:The role of illness-related and psycho-social factors.* Dissertation Abstracts International: Section B: The Sciences & Engineering, 65(3-B) 1564. US: University Microfilms International.

Thomas, V. J. & Taylor, L. M (2002). The Psychosocial experience of people with sickle cell disease and its impact on quality of life; Qualitative findings from focus group. *British Journal of Health Psychology* 7, 345-363.

Vichinsky, E. P., Neumayr, L. D., Gold, J. I., Weiner, M. W., Rule, R. R., Truran, D., et al., (2010). Neuropsychological Dysfunction and Neuroimaging Abnormalities in Neurologically Intact Adults With sickle cell anaemia. *JAMA*, 303(18), 1823-1831.

Wang, W. C. (2007). The pathophysiology, prevention, and treatment of stroke in *sickle cell* disease.*Current Opinion in Haematology*. 14, 191–197

Wasserman, A. L., Wilimas, J. A., Fairclough, D. L., Mulhern, R. K., & Wang, W. (1991).Subtle neuropsychological deficits in children with sickle cell disease. *The American Journal of Paediatric Haematology/ Oncology*, 13(1), 14-20.

Wilde, N. J., Strauss, E., & Tulsky, D. S. (2004). Memory Span on the Wechsler Scales. *Journal of Clinical Experimental Neuropsychology* 26, 539-549.

Chapter 12

Psychological Wellbeing and Quality of Life among Chronic Kidney Disease Patients in Ghana

Vincent Boima, Vincent Ganu, David Adjei, Charlotte Osafo, Michael Mate-Kole, Dwomoa Adu and C. Charles Mate-Kole

Introduction

Chronic kidney disease is rarely reversible and leads to a progressive decline in renal function. This occurs even after a precipitating event has been removed. End stage renal disease (ESRD) is the loss of renal function requiring treatment with chronic dialysis or transplantation.

The burden of chronic kidney disease (CKD) and the resulting ESRD is known worldwide (Coresh et al., 2007). Aside the high rate of morbidity and mortality associated with CKD, it presents with economic challenges (Cass et al., 2006).

Epidemiologic studies have indicated that the incidence of CKD is higher in developing countries than in the industrialized world (Remuzzi, 2001). Data are often not available in Africa either on the burden of CKD or on psychological wellbeing or on the quality of life of patients with the disease. According to Korle Bu Teaching Hospital records (the largest hospital in Ghana), about 15 percent of all medical admissions to the hospital are due to kidney disease, and the mortality rate of CKD is estimated at 10 percent. CKD is known to kill young Ghanaians between the ages of 20-50 years (Mate-Kole, Affram, Lee et al., 1993). Thus, many people in the economically active group of our society are being silently wiped out by this disease.

The cost of hemodialysis is US $ 100.00 per session in Ghana and the patient is required to undergo at least three sessions per week. The cost of additional medication further raises the cost of treatment, especially when there is limited access to transplantation surgery in the country. For a developing country like Ghana, the majority of the patients who need this treatment unfortunately cannot afford it.

CKD affects patients' overall functioning. The associated demands, including treatment, management and economic status have a significant impact on the patient's physical and psychological wellbeing and interfere with the patients' ability to cope with such a disabling illness. Patients with CKD, including those who are undergoing renal replacement therapy (RRT), often experience difficulties in participating in various domains of life, such as employment, social and leisure activities. The resulting psychological complications are profound. Psychological problems include depression, anxiety, fear, and emotional fluctuation; these changes are more pronounced especially at the early phase of the treatment. Thus, the patient's quality of life (QoL) is significantly compromised (Schieppati & Remuzzi, 2005).

This chapter will address psychological factors such as depression, quality of life, and cognitive consequences of chronic kidney disease and end-stage renal disease (ESRD).

Depression

The World Health Organization has highlighted depression as the second most common and economically costly chronic disease that will affect non-medically ill people globally over the next decades (Ustun, Ayuso-Mateos, Chatterji, et al., 2004). Depression in patients with other medical or psychiatric illness, is typically of greater intensity and more difficult to treat than depression occurring in patients without underlying disorders (Kimmel, 2001).

CKD is a progressive, life-threatening illness, posing fundamental psychological and social problems for individuals as well as a burden on their families. The interplay between the person's genetic susceptibility, his/her socioeconomic circumstances, and bio-psychosocial factors may trigger depression at any point of the disease process. On the psychological level, starting dialysis requires a complex emotional and cognitive-behavioral adaptation from patients. Individuals whose kidney functions decline rapidly or who are not aware of their illness until its final stage become suddenly and unexpectedly, "severely ill". Adults with CKD who used to take charge of their daily functioning become dependent on healthcare professionals and on their own family members to a significant degree. Unfortunately, research on the psychological impact of CKD, to our knowledge, is not available in Ghana. To date, we are aware of anecdotal reports which highlight the extent of this debilitating illness. We provide below, a case example of a patient after inception of dialysis:

Case - AB, a 60 year- old man diagnosed with ESRD due to longstanding high blood pressure. *He had all the financial resources and family support needed during therapy (significant because the majority of our cases do not usually have the financial resources to afford the treatment). On being informed of his condition and the limited treatment options, he became extremely hostile within the first week of dialysis and he refused to communicate with both healthcare providers at the dialysis unit and his caregivers at home. He was angry all the time. In addition, he refused to take his medication and meals. An interview with a relative revealed that this was a man who, prior to his illness, was in control of his life; he made decisions at home and work, and managed his affairs very well. However, with his current condition, he realized that he could no longer "be in charge". He was devastated and depressed with feelings of helplessness. AB was prescribed anti-depressants in addition to receiving emotional support. After three months, his dysphoric symptoms improved and he started communicating with the staff. Despite his good financial status, AB was not protected from the psychological complications of the disease.*

Risk factors for depression both in the general population and in CKD patients include unemployment, low income, and living alone (Lopes et al., 2004). Those chronic disease patients who require dialysis often have to give up their jobs. Although transplantation gives more independence to patients, the vocational activity level stays low and the majority of patients cannot afford the cost.

Since our patients in general receive hemodialysis, we would argue that depression may partly be linked to the treatment; the continuous connection to the hemodialysis machine during dialysis and the significant restrictions on independent living (Karamanidou et al., 2009; Kimmel & Peterson, 2005)).

Recent studies using gold-standard measurements have shown a prevalence of depression of 26–27 percent in the dialysis population (Hedayati, Bosworth, Kuchibhatla et al., 2006). This is in sharp contrast to the prevalence of major depressive disorder in the general population which is estimated at 5 percent.

Depression is characterized by both cognitive and somatic features. The somatic characteristics have an uncanny similarity to the symptoms of uremia, such as anorexia, sleep disturbances, fatigue, gastrointestinal disorders and pain (Kimmel, 2002; Kimmel & Peterson, 2005). This may sometimes make it difficult to diagnose depression in CKD patients; thus, one needs awareness of the clinical signs of depression. Overall, depression is largely under-diagnosed in CKD patients (Kimmel, 2002; Lopes et al., 2004). Furthermore, depression might cause differential outcomes (quality of life) in patients with ESRD through its effects, compliance, nutrition, immune status, marital and family dynamics, or through differential access to care (Kimmel & Peterson, 2005).

Lopes et al. (2002), using data from the large Dialysis Outcomes and Practice Patterns (DOPPS) study, reported that a diagnosis of depression or increased level of depressive affect was associated with increased morbidity and mortality in CKD patients. Knight and colleagues (Knight, Ofsthun, Teng et al., 2003), in a longitudinal study using Short Form 36 (SF-36) based measures, reported that the baseline Mental Component Score (mental health) assessed one to three months after initiating ESRD therapy with haemodialysis, revealed a declining score (lowered mental health) over time, which decline was significantly associated with high mortality.

The assessment of psychological distress in the earlier stages of CKD has been largely neglected. In a study conducted in a pre-dialysis clinic, approximately 50% of patients reported severe depressive symptoms (Walters, Hays, Spritzer et al., 2002). Overall, CKD, like most chronic diseases, can be regarded as a significant risk factor for major depression. Thus, there is the need for active intervention of depressive symptoms in CKD (Stewart, Ricci, Chee, et al., 2003).

Cognitive impairment

Another psychological component that requires attention in the treatment and management of CKD is cognitive impairment, which is a common occurrence, especially among patients with ESRD (Bremer, Wert, Durica, & Weaver, 1997). Cognitive deficits, including difficulties with concentration, memory and planning may hinder the patient's ability to participate in their own care, for example in terms of dietary modification, medication compliance, understanding of the rationale of treatment and appreciation of the complexities of medical procedures (Bremer et al., 1997). The mechanism for the cognitive deficits, although partially attributable to depression, may include other risk factors like uremia, complication of dialysis procedure and high prevalence of clinical and sub-clinical diseases such as hypertension, diabetes, malnutrition and co-morbid conditions associated with ESRD. Recent studies have shown that CKD is a risk factor for cognitive impairment (Kurella, Yaffe, Shlipak et al., 2005). In early asymptomatic stages of CKD, there is deficit in cerebral cognitive function. The data indicate that the decline in cognition occurs in a graded fashion from stages 3 to 4 then finally to 5 with severe dysfunction in the later stages of CKD (Madan, Kalra, Agarwal, & Tandon, 2007).

The risk of cognitive impairment and dementia in elderly patients with CKD is more than double that of the general population (Fukunishi et al., 2002). Elderly CKD patients have poorer performance on tests of global cognitive function, executive function, language and memory (Kurella et al., 2005). However, studies have shown an improvement in cognition after transplantation and after conversion from conventional hemodialysis to nocturnal dialysis (Jassal, Devins, Chan, Bozanovic, & Rourke, 2006). Therefore, it is reasonable to suggest that modifiable factors such as uremic toxins, fluid overload, and anemia amongst others associated with ESRD or its treatment may be the underlying pathogenesis of impaired cognition in these patients. Nevertheless it is known that moderate to severe cognitive impairment is common and undiagnosed in patients on hemodialysis (Murray et al., 2006).

Quality of life in chronic renal disease

Low quality of life, depression and other psychological problems tend to worsen the prognosis of CKD (Kalantar-Zadeh, Kopple, Block, et al., 2001). Quality of life may be described as a broad ranging concept affected in a complex way by the person's physical health, psychological state, level of independence, social relationships, and their relationships to salient features of their environment (Billington, 1999). In the mid-to-late 1970s, a predominant concern relating to QoL emphasized how health or its absence impacted the daily functioning of populations. This trend has become a critically important concept for health care and is categorized as a subset of QoL, which is broadly entitled health-related QoL (Suet-Ching, 2001). Health-related QoL has emerged as a conceptualization of health that can be measured and used as a quality indicator and as a concept, has drawn attention to the promotion of mental health (Christensen & Ehlers, 2002).

Despite a tremendous increase in knowledge and skills in the management of ESRD patients, such individuals, particularly those treated by hemodialysis, remain ill. They have impaired health-related QoL, dependence on others, and poor rehabilitation which may persist even in well-dialyzed ESRD patients (Mittal et al., 2001). It is recognized that regardless of the treatment method, patients suffering from ESRD have to cope with many adversities (e.g. physical symptoms, specific dietary regimes and changes in their body image), while their control over treatment cannot always be predicted (Mavromates, 2005). Such constraints are expected to affect the patients' quality of life leading patients to reconsider their personal and professional goals within the context of living with a chronic illness.

The traditional factors which predict good QoL include the following: age less than 65 years (Seica et al., 2009), hemoglobin levels less than 11.1g/dl (Abu-Alfa et al., 2008), urea reduction ratio greater than 65 percent (Lew & Patel, 2007), albumin greater than 40g/L(Owen, Lew, Liu, Lowrie, & Lazarus, 1993), the absence of co-morbidities, for example diabetes and hypertension (Spiegel, Melmed, Robbins, & Esrailian, 2008), higher socioeconomic and educational status (Mapes et al., 2004). Race also has an influence on QoL- black patients with ESRD in the United States (Owen, 1996) and Britain (Bakewell, Higgins, &

Edmunds, 2001) have demonstrated higher QoL scores than matched Caucasian patients despite having negative predictors of QoL.

In Ghana, only a small number of patients are on RRT (dialysis and kidney transplantation) due to the cost of dialysis and that of the surgery for the transplantation. The majority of ESRD patients cannot afford these treatment options, and thus are managed conservatively. Among the patients on dialysis, approximately 5-10 percent only are able to sustain this modality of treatment and therefore few enjoy the benefits of this treatment. Approximately 10 percent agree to have dialysis initially, and are able to raise funds to start the treatment. Nevertheless, with time, their sources of funds get exhausted and they are unable to continue the treatment or reduce the number of sessions required per week. As a result, although the average patient needs at least 3 sessions per week to feel well, most end up having two and/ or even one per week. In view of this, they are unable to achieve their optimal level; rather, they tend to have a poor quality of life.

Case example:

HT, 16 years old, was diagnosed with ESRD due to chronic glomerulonephritis. It was obvious from the onset that his parents could not afford renal replacement therapy. The clinical picture of this patient at this time was life threatening; without dialysis he would die. Fortunately, some visitors in our unit at the time from the United Kingdom attended one of our ward rounds. On seeing HT's condition, one of them decided to secure funds in the UK to support HT's dialysis and subsequent kidney transplantation. On account of this, dialysis was commenced immediately, and it revived him from a moribund state. His condition was improving when suddenly, his sponsors withdrew their support. Consequently his family could only afford dialysis at most, once a week. HT's condition deteriorated and he died. This is the clinical picture of almost about 30% of patients who visit the dialysis unit for treatment.

While renal replacement therapies can maintain patients indefinitely and prolong life, the quality of life is severely affected (de Francisco & Pinera, 2006). Renal transplantation increases the survival of patients with ESRD significantly when compared to other therapeutic options (Groothoff, 2005); however, it is associated with increased short-term mortality due to complications of the surgery. Transplantation aside, high-intensity home hemodialysis appears to be associated with improved survival and a greater quality of life, when compared to the conventional three times a week hemodialysis and peritoneal dialysis (Pierratos, McFarlane, & Chan, 2005).

It is known that health-related QoL is an independent risk factor for mortality in patients with ESRD (Simic-Ogrizovic et al., 2009). The relative risk of mortality in these patients ranges from 1.25 – 2.02 for each 10-point reduction in physical role and social functioning QoL domains (Kalantar-Zadeh et al., 2001).

Even though it is evident from various studies that ESRD patients tended to have a poorer QoL compared to the general population, it must be noted that most of these studies were cross-sectional and were small in size (Molsted, Prescott, Heaf, & Eidemak, 2007). In addition the larger studies lacked a longitudinal component (Perlman et al., 2005) and the longitudinal studies have been small in size as well (Gorodetskaya et al., 2005) and used tools that were not developed for patients with chronic kidney disease(Lash et al., 2006).

Overall, the majority of the studies were conducted in Europe and North America; thus the outcome may not necessarily be applicable in its entirety noting the cultural factors that can influence treatment outcome.

Future directions

As outlined in this chapter, chronic kidney disease (CKD) and the subsequent end-stage renal disease, is a debilitating condition which for a significant number of patients carries a death sentence. Psycho-social complications such as depression and compromised quality of life are additional factors that can impact the patient's treatment regimen, even allowing for those patients who can bear the financial burden of treatment. The psychosocial complications significantly affect the patient's morale, self-esteem and motivation to cope with the many facets of the condition.

It is reasonable therefore, to argue for a paradigm shift to include coping mechanisms as a part of a holistic approach to treatment. One such dimension is the role of spirituality and religiosity.

The areas of spirituality and/or religiosity have not been fully considered in the health-related QoL instruments until recently when focus groups around the world reported that spirituality affects QoL and that it should be considered an important component of health-related QoL (WHO, 1995). Spirituality encompasses participation in organized religious as well as existential beliefs, acknowledging a higher Being or power (Berman et al., 2004). Spirituality in the Ghanaian context is critical and the increasing attention to spiritual wellbeing is partly a result of associated benefits including psychosocial adjustment to the illness and lower use of health services (Koenig et al., 1999). It also involves the need for finding satisfactory answers to questions about the meaning of life, illness and death. Recent data support the importance of spirituality for CKD patients. Spirituality may be an important determinant of quality of life in CKD (Davison & Jhangri, 2010).

In Ghana, for example, people are highly religious and spiritual. For significant numbers of CKD patients, the first contact when they fall ill is either the traditional or the faith healer. The role of faith and beliefs in the life of Ghanaians is very important. Like Africans in general, the Ghanaian is a spiritual being and will ultimately, in the face of an illness or any dire consequences, ensure that they obtain spiritual fulfilment. Most of them spend time in faith homes, prayer camps, or traditional centers; some arrive in hospital when the disease is well advanced. Religious beliefs may give meaning, hope and comfort, even in situations of extreme suffering, by providing an explanation for the experience of illness and helping people to value themselves and their lives despite the illness. An estimate of one's meaningfulness of life is reported to be the most important resource in coping with an illness as it motivates people to adopt other coping strategies (Antonovsky, 1987). Consequently, targeting spirituality in ESRD patients may help to preserve or enhance health-related QoL even in the face of considerable physical and psychosocial challenges.

Conclusions

The role of psychological therapies for renal patients is becoming increasingly important due to the problems outlined earlier. ESRD patients are at risk of depression; thus the role of psychological intervention cannot be overstated; in fact, it is long overdue. There is the need for a more holistic approach to the treatment and management of the chronic renal patient. This multidisciplinary approach should involve mental health professionals like clinical psychologists and psychiatrists. In addition, the role of pastoral counselors and sources for spiritual relief should be considered, bearing in mind that the African is a spiritual and religious being.

CKD patients should have early psychological and cognitive assessment in addition to ensuring their spiritual needs are met. Psychological counseling may then be started early to prepare the patient to better cope with a lifelong illness.

Patients and their caregivers require in-depth counseling at the onset of their illness and before the inception of RRT. These counseling sessions should clearly outline the nature and course of the disease, treatment options (including cost of treatment) and prognosis. We would argue that a holistic approach to the treatment, care and management of the chronic kidney disease patient in Ghana is urgently needed.

References

Antonovsky A., (1987). *Unraveling the Mystery of Health,* London:John Bass Publishers.

Abu-Alfa, A. K., Sloan, L., Charytan, C., Sekkarie, M., Scarlata, D., Globe, D., & Audhya, P. (2008). The association of darbepoetin alfa with hemoglobin and health-related quality of life in patients with chronic kidney disease not receiving dialysis. *Curr Med Res Opin, 24*(4), 1091-1100.

Bakewell, A. B., Higgins, R. M., & Edmunds, M. E. (2001). Does ethnicity influence perceived quality of life of patients on dialysis and following renal transplant? *Nephrol Dial Transplant, 16*(7), 1395-1401.

Berman, E., Merz, J. F., Rudnick, M., Snyder, R. W., Rogers, K. K., Lee, J. & Lipschutz, J. H. (2004). Religiosity in a hemodialysis population and its relationship to satisfaction with medical care, satisfaction with life, and adherence. *Am J Kidney Dis, 44*(3), 488-497.

Billington DR. (1999) WHOQOL Annotated Bibliography.:Geneva, World Health Organization.

Bremer, B. A., Wert, K. M., Durica, A. L., & Weaver, A. (1997). Neuropsychological, physical, and psychosocial functioning of individuals with end-stage renal disease. [Research Support, Non-US Gov't]. *Ann Behav Med, 19*(4), 348-352.

Cass, A., Chadban, S., Craig, J., Howard, K., McDonald, S., Salkeld, G., & White, S. (2006). *The economic impact of end-stage kidney disease in Australia.*Melbourne: Kidney Health Australia.

Christensen, A. J., & Ehlers, S. L. (2002). Psychological factors in end-stage renal disease: an emerging context for behavioral medicine research. [Research Support, US Gov't PHS Review]. *J Consult Clin Psychol, 70*(3), 712-724.

Coresh, J., Selvin, E., Stevens, L. A., Manzi, J., Kusek, J. W., Eggers, P., Levey, A. S. (2007). Prevalence of chronic kidney disease in the United States. [Research Support, N I H , Extramural]. *Jama, 298*(17), 2038-2047. doi: 10.1001/jama.298.17.2038

Davison, S. N., & Jhangri, G. S. (2010). Existential and supportive care needs among patients with chronic kidney disease. *J Pain Symptom Manage, 40*(6), 838-843.

De Francisco, A. L., & Pinera, C. (2006). Challenges and future of renal replacement therapy. *Hemodial Int, 10*(1), S19-23.

Fukunishi, I., Kitaoka, T., Shirai, T., Kino, K., Kanematsu, E., & Sato, Y. (2002). Psychiatric disorders among patients undergoing hemodialysis therapy. *Nephron, 91*(2), 344-347.

Gorodetskaya, I., Zenios, S., McCulloch, C. E., Bostrom, A., Hsu, C. Y., Bindman, A. B. & Chertow, G. M. (2005). Health-related quality of life and estimates of utility in chronic kidney disease. *Kidney Int, 68*(6), 2801-2808.

Groothoff, J. W. (2005). Long-term outcomes of children with end-stage renal disease.*Pediatr Nephrol, 20*(7), 849-853.

Hedayati, S. S., Bosworth, H. B., Kuchibhatla, M., Kimmel, P. L., & Szczech, L. A. (2006). The predictive value of self-report scales compared with physician diagnosis of depression in hemodialysis patients. . *Kidney Int, 69*(9), 1662-1668.

Jassal, S. V., Devins, G. M., Chan, C. T., Bozanovic, R., & Rourke, S. (2006). Improvements in cognition in patients converting from thrice weekly hemodialysis to nocturnal hemodialysis: a longitudinal pilot study. *Kidney Int, 70*(5), 956-962.

Kalantar-Zadeh, K., Kopple, J. D., Block, G., & Humphreys, M. H. (2001). Association among SF36 quality of life measures and nutrition, hospitalization, and mortality in hemodialysis. *J Am Soc Nephrol, 12*(12), 2797-2806.

Karamanidou C, T. P., Ginieri-Coccossis M et al. (2009). Anxiety, depression and health beliefs in end-stage renal disease (ESRD) patients. *In: Proceedings of the 17th European Congress of Psychiatry, Lisbon, Portugal, abstract R38.*

Kimmel, P. L. (2001). Psychosocial factors in dialysis patients. *Kidney Int, 59*(4), 1599-1613.

Kimmel, P. L. (2002). Depression in patients with chronic renal disease: what we know and what we need to know. *J Psychosom Res, 53*(4), 951-956.

Kimmel, P. L., & Peterson, R. A. *Depression in patients with end-stage renal disease treated with dialysis: has the time to treat arrived? In : Clin J Am Soc Nephrol.* 2006 May;1(3):349-52. Epub 2006 Apr 12.

Kimmel, P. L., & Peterson, R. A. (2005). Depression in end-stage renal disease patients treated with hemodialysis: tools, correlates, outcomes, and needs. *Semin Dial, 18*(2), 91-97.

Knight, E. L., Ofsthun, N., Teng, M., Lazarus, J. M., & Curhan, G. C. (2003). The association between mental health, physical function, and hemodialysis mortality. *Kidney Int, 63*(5), 1843-1851.

Koenig, H. G., Idler, E., Kasl, S., Hays, J. C., George, L. K., Musick, M., Benson, H. *Religion, spirituality, and medicine: a rebuttal to skeptics*: Int J Psychiatry Med. 1999;29(2):123-31.

Kurella, M., Yaffe, K., Shlipak, M. G., Wenger, N. K., & Chertow, G. M. (2005). Chronic kidney disease and cognitive impairment in menopausal women.. *Am J Kidney Dis, 45*(1), 66-76.

Lash, J. P., Wang, X., Greene, T., Gadegbeku, C. A., Hall, Y., Jones, K., Unruh, M. (2006). Quality of life in the African American Study of Kidney Disease and Hypertension: effects of blood pressure management. . *Am J Kidney Dis, 47*(6), 956-964.

Levy, J., Brown, E., Daley, C., & Lawrence, A. (2009). *Oxford Handbook of dialysis*: NEW York: Oxford University Press.

Lew, S. Q., & Patel, S. S. (2007). Psychosocial and quality of life issues in women with end-stage renal disease. . *Adv Chronic Kidney Dis, 14*(4), 358-363.

Lopes, A. A., Albert, J. M., Young, E. W., Satayathum, S., Pisoni, R. L., Andreucci, V. E., Port, F. K. (2004). Screening for depression in hemodialysis patients: associations with diagnosis, treatment, and outcomes in the DOPPS. *Kidney Int, 66*(5), 2047-2053.

Lopes, A. A., Bragg, J., Young, E., Goodkin, D., Mapes, D., Combe, C., Port, F. K. (2002). Depression as a predictor of mortality and hospitalization among hemodialysis patients in the United States and Europe. *Kidney Int, 62*(1), 199-207.

Madan, P., Kalra, O. P., Agarwal, S., & Tandon, O. P. (2007). Cognitive impairment in chronic kidney disease. *Nephrol Dial Transplant, 22*(2), 440-444.

Mapes, D. L., Bragg-Gresham, J. L., Bommer, J., Fukuhara, S., McKevitt, P., Wikstrom, B., & Lopes, A. A. (2004). Health-related quality of life in the Dialysis Outcomes and Practice Patterns Study (DOPPS). *Am J Kidney Dis, 44*(5 Suppl 2), 54-60.

Mate-Kole, M., Affram, K., Lee, S. J., Howie, A. J., Michael, J., & Adu, D. (1993). Hypertension and end-stage renal failure in tropical Africa. *J Hum Hypertens, 7*(5), 443-446.

Mittal, S. K., Ahern, L., Flaster, E., Mittal, V. S., Maesaka, J. K., & Fishbane, S. (2001). Self-assessed quality of life in peritoneal dialysis patients. *Am J Nephrol, 21*(3), 215-220.

Molsted, S., Prescott, L., Heaf, J., & Eidemak, I. (2007). Assessment and clinical aspects of health-related quality of life in dialysis patients and patients with chronic kidney disease. *Nephron Clin Pract, 106*(1), c24-33.

Murray, A. M., Tupper, D. E., Knopman, D. S., Gilbertson, D. T., Pederson, S. L., Li, S., . . . Nilsson, J., Rana, A. K., & Kabir, Z. N. (2006). Social capital and quality of life in old age: results from a cross-sectional study in rural Bangladesh. *J Aging Health, 18*(3), 419-434.

Owen, W. F., Jr. (1996). Racial differences in incidence, outcome, and quality of life for African-Americans on hemodialysis. [Comparative Study]. *Blood Purif, 14*(4), 278-285.

Owen, W. F., Jr., Lew, N. L., Liu, Y., Lowrie, E. G., & Lazarus, J. M. (1993). The urea reduction ratio and serum albumin concentration as predictors of mortality in patients undergoing hemodialysis. *N Engl J Med, 329*(14), 1001-1006.

Perlman, R. L., Finkelstein, F. O., Liu, L., Roys, E., Kiser, M., Eisele, G., Saran, R. (2005). Quality of life in chronic kidney disease (CKD): a cross-sectional analysis in the Renal Research Institute-CKD study. *Am J Kidney Dis, 45*(4), 658-666.

Pierratos, A., McFarlane, P., & Chan, C. T. (2005). Quotidian dialysis--update 2005. *Curr Opin Nephrol Hypertens, 14*(2), 119-124.

Remuzzi G., (July 2001). A research program for COMGAN. ISN News. 1–6.

Schieppati, A., & Remuzzi, G. (2005). Chronic renal diseases as a public health problem: epidemiology, social, and economic implications. *Kidney Int Suppl, 98*, S7-S10.

Seica, A., Segall, L., Verzan, C., Vaduva, N., Madincea, M., Rusoiu, S., Covic, A. (2009). Factors affecting the quality of life of haemodialysis patients from Romania: a multicentric study. *Nephrol Dial Transplant, 24*(2), 626-629.

Simic-Ogrizovic, S., Jemcov, T., Pejanovic, S., Stosovic, M., Radovic, M., & Djukanovic, L. (2009). Health-related quality of life, treatment efficacy, and hemodialysis patient outcome. *Ren Fail, 31*(3), 201-206.

Spiegel, B. M., Melmed, G., Robbins, S., & Esrailian, E. (2008). Biomarkers and health-related quality of life in end-stage renal disease: a systematic review. *Clin J Am Soc Nephrol, 3*(6), 1759-1768.

Stewart, W. F., Ricci, J. A., Chee, E., Hahn, S. R., & Morganstein, D. (2003). Cost of lost productive work time among US workers with depression. *Jama, 289*(23), 3135-3144.

Suet-Ching, W. L. (2001). The psychometric properties of the Chinese Dialysis Quality of Life Scale for Hong Kong dialysis patients. . *J Adv Nurs, 36*(3), 441-449.

Ustun, T. B., Ayuso-Mateos, J. L., Chatterji, S., Mathers, C., & Murray, C. J. (2004). Global burden of depressive disorders in the year 2000. *Br J Psychiatry, 184*, 386-392.

Vazquez, I., Valderrabano, F., Fort, J., Jofre, R., Lopez-Gomez, J. M., Moreno, F., & Sanz-Guajardo, D. (2005). Psychosocial factors and health-related quality of life in hemodialysis patients.*Qual Life Res, 14*(1), 179-190.

Walters, B. A., Hays, R. D., Spritzer, K. L., Fridman, M., & Carter, W. B. (2002). Health-related quality of life, depressive symptoms, anemia, and malnutrition at hemodialysis initiation. *Am J Kidney Dis, 40*(6), 1185-1194.

World Health Organization (1995) The World Health Organization Quality of Life assessment (WHOQOL): position paper from the World Health Organization. *Soc Sci Med, 41*(10), 1403-1409.

Chapter 13

Irritable Bowel Syndrome and related Functional Bowel Disorders in an Urban Gastroenterology Practice

Timothy N. A. Archampong and K. N. Nkrumah,

Introduction

Functional bowel disorders (FBDs) are defined by several combinations of persistent and fluctuating gastrointestinal symptoms without an identifiable organic basis following clinical and investigative assessments. Irritable bowel syndrome (IBS), an FBD, is a gastrointestinal syndrome characterized by chronic abdominal pain and altered bowel habit in the absence of any organic cause (Drossman et al., 1993). It is the most commonly diagnosed gastrointestinal condition (Drossman, et al., 1993). The prevalence of IBS in North America and Europe estimated from population-based studies is approximately 10-15% (Drossman, et al., 1993). Its prevalence among Kenyans attending an urban private hospital was 8% with sufferers predominantly in the 3rd decade of life (Lule & Amayo, 2002). Its comparative prevalence in industrialised countries suggests that irritable bowel syndrome is not a rare clinical condition in Africa. A community-based study in western Nigeria showed a prevalence rate of 30% for IBS among students, reflecting a differing distribution of disease (Lule & Amayo, 2002). Information is, however, limited on the trends of other functional diseases in Africa.

IBS affects men and women, young patients, and the elderly. However, younger patients and women are more likely to be diagnosed with IBS. A systematic review estimated that there is an overall 2:1 female predominance in North America (Brandt et al., 2009). Other populations may have differing epidemiologic features: Several population-based studies from Asia showed that the frequency of functional dyspepsia was not related to gender (Kwan et al., 2003). However IBS was more common among males in Jos, Nigeria, with

52.9% males (Okeke et al., 2009). Socio-cultural and lifestyle factors vary across populations and tend to influence expression and severity of functional bowel diseases. Ethnicity and dietary factors have also been implicated, including the gastro-intestinal sensitivity to peppery foods and carbohydrate-based diets. The cause of functional bowel disorders is not definitive; hence there is no discrete lesion to be targeted therapeutically (Sainsbury & Ford, 2011). Soluble fibre and antispasmodics have been shown to improve symptoms, however, individual responses are variable (Bijkerk et al., 2009). Antidepressants also appear to be more effective than placebo in treating IBS patients (Drossman et al., 2010). This report describes current concepts of the clinical expression and management of the prevalent FBDs, IBS and non-ulcer dyspepsia (NUD), highlighting lifestyle factors and specific management strategies in the Ghanaian setting.

Irritable bowel syndrome: a review of observational data in KBTH, Accra

Clinical information was collated from medical records of new and follow-up patients attending the Gastroenterology Unit of the Korle Bu Teaching Hospital (KBTH), Accra, between February 2002 and March, 2012 for suspected functional bowel disorders.

Korle Bu Teaching Hospital is the main tertiary referral centre in Accra serving the majority of the southern half of Ghana. The Gastro-enterology Unit runs a weekly afternoon Outpatient Clinic and is the principal referral centre for gastro-intestinal diseases in Southern Ghana. Approximately 50 patients attend each clinic session. The study survey was structured with specific questions to identify all patients with functional bowel disease as stated in the Rome III diagnostic criteria (Drossman et al., 2010) and to capture response to therapy. One-hundred and seventy-five (175) case files with gastroenterological conditions were reviewed, excluding liver-related diseases. The FBD review yielded 125 patients of which 52.8 percent (66) were males and 47.2 percent (59) females. The male-female ratio of patients with functional bowel disease of 1.12: 1 was similar to the result obtained from the prevalence of irritable bowel syndrome in a Nigerian study and contrary to Western countries where the female-male ratio appears to be higher (Chang, 2004). This may suggest a different pattern of illness behaviour in Ghanaians presenting with functional bowel disease. The mean age was 39.83 years, higher than other comparative studies in Africa (Ladep, Obindo, Audu, Okeke, & Malu, 2006).

The youngest being 10 and the oldest 55 years. Irritable bowel syndrome (IBS) 36.8 percent (n: 45) was the most prevalent in comparison to non-ulcer dyspepsia (NUD) (34.4 percent (n: 43), functional diarrhoea 4.8 percent (n: 6), functional constipation 3.2 percent (n: 4), functional heartburn 3.2 percent (n: 4), functional abdominal pain syndrome 8 percent (n: 10), unexplained excessive belching 1.6 percent (n: 2) and unexplained abdominal pain 8 percent (n: 10). The majority of our cases were either non-ulcer dyspepsia (34.4%) or irritable bowel syndrome (36%) as reported in other studies (Dobrek & Thor, 2009). Non-ulcer dyspepsia had a high prevalence in this descriptive study; similar to other European studies (Hirakawa et al., 1999).

Pathophysiology

The etiology of IBS and FBD is expressed by a myriad of suspected patho-physiological mechanisms as no clear cause-effect exists in its genesis.

Gastro-intestinal motility: Abnormalities observed include increased frequency and irregularity of gastrointestinal contractions, prolonged transit time in constipation-predominant IBS, and an exaggerated motor response to cholecystokinin and meal ingestion in diarrhea-predominant IBS (Chey, Jin, Lee, Sun, & Lee, 2001). The pharmacological stimulation of gut motility in IBS patients has been shown to reduce luminal gas and improve symptoms, suggesting that a dys-motility syndrome precipitates IBS in some patients (Caldarella, Serra, Azpiroz, & Malagelada, 2002).

Visceral hypersensitivity: Visceral hypersensitivity (increased sensation in response to stimuli) is a frequent finding in IBS patients. Perception in the gastrointestinal (GI) tract results from stimulation of various receptors in the gut wall. These receptors transmit signals via afferent neural pathways to the dorsal horn of the spinal cord and ultimately to the brain. Studies have focused on selective hyper-sensitization of visceral afferent nerves in the gut, triggered by bowel distension, as a possible explanation for IBS. Studies report that in patients with IBS, awareness and pain caused by balloon distention in the gut are experienced at lower balloon volumes compared with controls, suggesting receptor hypersensitivity. Rectal distension in patients with IBS also triggered more cerebral cortical activity than in controls. However, in one study involving balloon distension of the descending colon, increased colonic sensitivity was influenced by a psychological tendency to report pain and urgency, rather than increased neuro-sensory sensitivity (Dorn et al., 2007).

Psychosocial dysfunction: Psychosocial factors influence the expression of IBS. In a study of patients with IBS, patients with GI symptoms reported more lifetime and daily stressful events than control groups (Locke, Weaver, Melton, & Talley, 2004). Another study found that, compared with controls, patients with IBS exhibit increased anxiety, depression, phobias, and somatisation (Solmaz, Kavuk, & Sayar, 2003). The role of stress in IBS is thought to be based upon corticotrophin releasing factor (CRF), a peptide released from the para-ventricular nucleus and considered to be a major mediator of the stress response. Data suggest that over-activity in the brain CRF and CRF-receptor signaling system contributes to anxiety disorders, IBS and depression (Keck & Holsboer, 2001).

Post-infectious IBS: Two meta-analyses demonstrated an increased risk of IBS in patients who experienced an episode of acute gastroenteritis (Thabane, Kottachchi, & Marshall, 2007). The increased risk of post-infectious IBS is associated with bacterial, protozoan, helminth infections, and viral infections. Specific bacterial pathogens included escherichia coli O157:H7 and campylobacter jejuni. A larger review reported that the odds of developing IBS are increased six-fold after an acute GI infection. Risk factors for post-infectious IBS include young age, prolonged fever, anxiety and depression (Thabane, et al., 2007) thereby emphasizing its inter-play with psychosocial factors.

Alteration in faecal micro-flora: The complex colonic micro-flora has led to speculation that changes in its composition could be associated with IBS. Emerging data suggest that the faecal micro-biota in individuals with IBS differ from healthy controls and vary with the predominant symptom (Kassinen et al., 2007). Additional studies are however needed to validate these observations. In view of potential micro-flora alterations in IBS, it is possible that patients with diarrhea-predominant IBS would benefit from probiotics, which influence the composition and metabolism of the micro-flora.

Dietary hypersensitivity and mal-absorption: The role of food in the patho-physiology of IBS is uncertain. Some patients with IBS report worsening of symptoms after eating specific foods and perceive intolerance to certain foods. Multiple factors have been considered to contribute to food sensitivity in patients with IBS, however studies reporting intolerance to specific foods by skin prick testing have been conflicting. One theoretical etiology of IBS suggests that symptoms may be related to impaired absorption of carbohydrates. The theory holds that fermentable oligo-, di-, and monosaccharides and polyols (FODMAPs) in patients with IBS or IBD enter the distal small bowel and colon where they are fermented, leading to symptoms and increased intestinal permeability and possibly inflammation. Fructose intolerance has been suggested as a possible form of carbohydrate mal-absorption contributing to GI symptoms such as flatus, pain, bloating, belching and altered bowel habits. Another study found that dietary restriction of fructose improved symptoms in patients with IBS who had been selected because of prior response to dietary change (Shepherd, Parker, Muir, & Gibson, 2008). Data suggest a similar absorption capacity of fructose, sorbitol and lactose in IBS patients and controls but symptoms occur more readily after a carbohydrate challenge in IBS.

Genetics: Familial studies and studies on select gene polymorphisms suggest a genetic susceptibility in some patients with IBS. Data from studies of twins are contradictory; some studies show a higher concordance rate for IBS in monozygotic twins compared with dizygotic twins while others have shown similar or comparable rates between these groups (Levy et al., 2001). In addition, another study found that having a parent with IBS was a greater independent predictor of IBS than having an affected twin, suggesting that the familial nature of IBS could be due to nurture as well as genetics (Levy, et al., 2001).

Clinical features

In the absence of a unifying etiological agent, efforts have been made to standardize the diagnosis of irritable bowel syndrome (IBS) using symptom-based criteria.

- Manning criteria: This concept originated in 1978 when Manning et al. formulated a symptom complex suggestive of IBS. These symptoms included relief of pain with bowel movements, increased stool consistency and frequency with onset of pain, passage of mucus, and a sense of incomplete emptying. There have been conflicting data regarding the predictive ability of the Manning criteria.

Table 13.1: Manning criteria for the diagnosis of irritable bowel syndrome*

Pain relieved with defecation
More frequent stools at the onset of pain
Looser stools at the onset of pain
Visible abdominal distention
Passage of mucus
Sensation of incomplete evacuation

** The likelihood of irritable bowel syndrome is proportional to the number of Manning criteria that are present.*

- Rome criteria: In an effort to standardize clinical research protocols, an international working team published a consensus definition in 1992 called the Rome criteria, which was revised most recently in 2005. IBS was defined as recurrent abdominal pain or discomfort associated with altered defecation.
- Supportive symptoms not part of the Rome III criteria include: abnormal stool frequency (≤3 bowel movements per week or >3 bowel movements per day), abnormal stool form (lumpy/hard or loose/watery), defecation straining, urgency, or a feeling of incomplete bowel movement, passing mucus and bloating.

Table 13.2: Rome III diagnostic criteria* for irritable bowel syndrome

Recurrent abdominal pain or discomfort• at least 3 days per month in the last 3 months associated with 2 or more of the following:
(1) Improvement with defecation
(2) Onset associated with a change in frequency of stool
(3) Onset associated with a change in form (appearance) of stool

** Criteria fulfilled for the last 3 months with symptom onset at least 6 months prior to diagnosis.*
• Discomfort means an uncomfortable sensation not described as pain.

Four subtypes of IBS have been identified epidemiologically:

- IBS with constipation (hard or lumpy stools ≥25 percent / loose or watery stools <25 percent of bowel movements);
- IBS with diarrhea (loose or water stools ≥25 percent / hard or lumpy stools <25 percent of bowel movements);
- Mixed IBS (hard or lumpy stools ≥25 percent / loose or watery stools ≥25 percent of bowel movements);
- Unsub-typed IBS (insufficient abnormality of stool consistency to meet the above subtypes).

Irritable bowel syndrome (IBS) can be identified by a variety of gastrointestinal and extra-intestinal complaints. However, the symptom complex of chronic abdominal pain and altered bowel habits remains the nonspecific yet primary characteristic of IBS.

Chronic abdominal pain: abdominal pain in IBS is usually described as a crampy colicky-type sensation with variable intensity in a fluctuating periodic fashion. The location and character of the pain can vary significantly. The severity of the pain may also range from a mild discomfort to crippling abdominal pain prompting an emergency unit visit. Several factors, such as emotional stress and eating specific foods, may exacerbate the pain, while defecation often provides some relief. At the Gastroenterology Clinic, 91% of patients with IBS had abdominal pain (n=45). Despite the variability of abdominal pain in IBS, some clinical features are not compatible with it and should alert the clinician to other structural GI disorders. These include pain associated with anorexia or weight loss. Although unlikely in IBS, they may imply a co-existing significant psychological illness such as depression. Pain that is progressive, awakens the patient from sleep, or prevents sleep is also unlikely to be IBS.

Change in Bowel Habit: Patients with IBS complain of an alteration in bowel function with all stool consistency scores reported; from diarrhea, constipation, alternating diarrhea and constipation, or normal bowel habits alternating with either diarrhea and/or constipation.

- Diarrhea: Diarrhea is usually characterized as frequent loose stools of small to moderate volume stool and occasional fecal incontinence. Stools generally occur during waking hours, most often in the morning or after meals. Most bowel movements are preceded by lower abdominal cramps and may be followed by a feeling of incomplete evacuation described as tenesmus. Approximately one-half of all patients with IBS complain of mucus discharge with stools (Manning, Thompson, Heaton, & Morris, 1978). At the GI Clinic, 17 of the 45 patients with IBS had predominant diarrhea with 29% complaining of additional mucus in the stool. Large volume diarrhea, bloody stools, nocturnal diarrhea, steatorrhoea are all associated with organic GI disease. A subgroup of IBS patients have symptoms immediately following an acute viral or bacterial, post-infectious IBS.
- Constipation: Constipation may be chronic or fluctuate with diarrhea or normal bowel habit. Stools are often hard and may be associated with tenesmus. This was reported in 27% of IBS patients at the GI Clinic.

Associated gastrointestinal symptoms: Upper gastrointestinal symptoms, including gastro-oesophageal reflux, dysphagia, early satiety, intermittent dyspepsia, nausea, and non-cardiac chest pain, are common in patients with IBS. Non-ulcer (functional) dyspepsia was present in 34.4% (n=43) of FBD patients in the GI Clinic, Patients with IBS also frequently complain of abdominal bloating and increased gas production in the form of flatulence or belching; these were reported in 51% of IBS patients reviewed in KBTH, Accra.

Extra-intestinal symptoms: Patients with IBS often complain of a broad range of non-gastrointestinal symptoms. These include impaired sexual function, dysmenorrhea, dyspareunia, increased urinary frequency and urgency, and fibromyalgia symptoms. In Accra, IBS patients reported a wide range of symptoms including recurrent coryzal symptoms, malaise (malaria-like symptoms) headaches, myalgia, arthralgia, insomnia, lethargy and palpitations. Also of interest were altered body sensations to taste and touch. Observational data collated at the Gastroenterology Clinic, Korle-Bu Teaching Hospital revealed the commonest reported extra-intestinal symptoms were headaches and generalized muscle aches in 20% and 24% of IBS patients respectively.

Irritable bowel syndrome: clinical precipitants in Accra: a comparative review

Hunger was a statistically significant precipitant in patients with NUD (p=0.0001). This raises the possibility of acid hyper-sensitivity as a potential patho-physiological mechanism in our patients. Tables 13.3 and 13.4 summarize the factors precipitating exacerbation of symptoms in the major functional bowel disorders (IBS/NUD). The role of diet in IBS has not been studied extensively, partly due to the diversity of dietary habits within populations. In the Gastroenterology Clinic study, the association between carbohydrate-based foods and irritable bowel syndrome was significant but no significant relationships were demonstrated between stress, smoking, beans, dairy food, spicy or carbonated drinks. The link between carbohydrates and IBS symptom-exacerbations may suggest selective carbohydrate mal-absorption as possible patho-physiological mechanisms in its expression locally.

In Asia, rice-based foods were better tolerated than Western diet in IBS sufferers (Wahnschaffe, Schulzke, Zeitz, & Ullrich, 2007). Spicy, peppery foods were prominent precipitants in Thailand (Gonlachanvit, Fongkam, Wittayalertpanya, & Kullavanijaya, 2007) and Malaysia (Mahadeva, Yadav, Rampal, Everett, & Goh, 2010). Alcohol use, was an important factor in tertiary care here in Accra as 30 percent of patients seen with IBS were drinkers (p=0.006). In the UK primary care setting, patients were more likely to be regular alcohol drinkers in comparison to a referred group (Longstreth et al., 2001). In our study population, smoking and alcohol did not achieve an association with non-ulcer dyspepsia as seen with peptic ulcer disease (Kang et al., 2011). This was similar to other population-based surveys of functional dyspepsia (Mahadeva & Goh, 2006). On the contrary, studies from the US, Europe and Asia have shown a risk association between smoking and alcohol for uninvestigated dyspepsia (Bernersen, Johnsen, & Straume, 1996).

Table 13.3: Factors associated with disease exacerbation in IBS

Precipitating factor	*IBS (%)	• Non-IBS (%)	**Total (n)	P value
Hunger	(20.0%)	(80.0%)	20	0.098
Stress	(60.0%)	(40.0%)	10	0.104
Spicy/peppery food	(54.5%)	(45.5%)	11	0.187
Carbohydrates	**(70.0%)**	**(30.0%)**	**10**	**0.021**
Dairy foods	(66.7%)	(33.3%)	6	0.113
Beans	(44.4%)	(55.6%)	9	0.597
Alcohol intake	(66.7%)	(33.3%)	21	0.006

**Proportion of IBS patients experiencing exacerbations with precipitant*

• Proportion of Non-IBS patients experiencing exacerbations with precipitant

***Total number of patients reporting symptom exacerbations with precipitant*

Table 13.4: Factors associated with disease exacerbation in NUD

Precipitating factor	*NUD (%)	• Non-NUD (%)	**Total (n)	P value
Hunger	**(75.0%)**	**(25.0%)**	**20**	**0.0001**
Spicy/peppery food	(9.1%)	(90.9%)	11	0.062
Stress	(20.0%)	(80.0%)	10	0.309
Carbohydrates	(20.0%)	(80.0%)	10	0.309
Dairy foods	(0%)	(100.0%)	6	0.067
Beans	(22.2%)	(77.8%)	9	0.415
Alcohol intake	(19.0%)	(81.0%)	21	0.112

**Proportion of NUD patients experiencing exacerbations with precipitant*

• Proportion of Non-NUD patients experiencing exacerbations with precipitant

***Total number of patients reporting symptom exacerbations with precipitant*

Management

The diagnostic approach:

The diagnosis of IBS and related FBDs is based upon the identification of positive symptoms consistent with the condition as summarized by the Rome criteria and excluding in a cost-effective manner other conditions with similar clinical presentations. Routine laboratory studies (full blood count, blood urea and electrolytes) are normal in IBS. Red flag features which are not compatible with IBS include rectal bleeding, nocturnal or progressive abdominal pain, weight loss, laboratory abnormalities such as anemia, elevated inflammatory markers, or electrolyte disturbances (Brandt, et al., 2009). Patients with any of these alarm symptoms required further imaging studies and/or colonoscopy. In patients who have symptoms suggestive of IBS, no alarm symptoms and no family history of inflammatory bowel disease or colorectal cancer, a limited number of diagnostic studies can rule out organic illness in the majority of patients. This limited diagnostic approach rules out organic disease in over 95 percent of patients.

The diagnostic evaluation depends upon whether the predominant symptom is diarrhea or constipation. In patients with diarrhea as the predominant symptom, stool cultures and colonoscopy will exclude infectious or inflammatory conditions. In patients with constipation as the predominant symptom or mixed IBS, a barium enema or flexible sigmoidoscopy/ colonoscopy will exclude a structural or obstructive lesion.

Irritable bowel syndrome: therapeutic options:

Irritable bowel syndrome (IBS) is a chronic condition therefore the focus of treatment should be on relief of symptoms and addressing the patient's concerns. Identifying recent exacerbating factors (e.g. medications, dietary changes), concerns about serious illness, stressors and psycho-social factors are essential when developing the optimum therapy.

Therapeutic relationship — The most important component of treatment lies in the establishment of a therapeutic physician-patient relationship. The doctor should be non-judgmental, establish realistic expectations with consistent limits and involve the patient in decision-making. Patients with established, positive physician interactions have fewer IBS-related follow-up visits.

Patient education — Education of the proposed mechanisms of IBS helps to validate the patient's illness experience and sets the basis for therapeutic interventions. Patients should be informed of the chronic and benign nature of IBS, and that he or she should have a normal life span.

Dietary modification — A careful dietary history may reveal patterns of symptoms related to specific foods. Given the similarity that may occur in symptoms of IBS and lactose intolerance, an empiric trial of a lactose-free diet should be considered in patients suspected of having irritable bowel syndrome (Bohmer & Tuynman, 2001). Some patients diagnosed with irritable bowel syndrome may have undiagnosed lactose intolerance and can have lasting clinical improvement when placed on a lactose-restricted diet (Bohmer & Tuynman, 2001).

Exclusion of foods that increase flatulence (beans, onions, carrots, raisins, bananas, prunes, yam) should be considered in patients who complain of gas.

Avoidance of carbohydrates has gained prominence as a dietary modification strategy in reducing symptoms in IBS (Gibson & Shepherd, 2005) but there have been few recent studies. Fructose intolerance has been suggested as a possible form of carbohydrate malabsorption contributing to IBS (Choi, Johlin, Summers, Jackson, & Rao, 2003). While diets low in FODMAPS have not been definitively shown to be of benefit, it is considered reasonable for refractory IBS patients to undergo a therapeutic trial of a low FODMAPS diet, provided that their nutritional status is being monitored. An increase in the intake of fiber is often recommended, either through diet or the use of commercial bulking supplements.

Psychosocial therapies — Behavioral treatments may be considered for motivated patients who associate symptoms with psycho-social stressors. Hypnosis, biofeedback, and psychotherapy help to reduce anxiety levels, encourage health promoting behaviour, increase patient responsibility and involvement in treatment, and improve pain tolerance (Brandt et al., 2009).

Irritable Bowel Syndrome: Pharmacological agents

Medications are only an adjunct to treatment in irritable bowel syndrome (IBS). Furthermore, the drug chosen varies depending on the patient's predominant symptoms. The chronic use of drugs is generally minimized or avoided because of the lifelong nature of this disorder, the lack of convincing long-term therapeutic benefit, variable outcomes and potential safety issues with some medications.

Antispasmodic agents — Antispasmodic agents are the most frequently used agents in the treatment of IBS. Certain antispasmodic drugs (hyoscine, cimetropium, and pinaverium) may provide short-term relief but long-term efficacy has not been demonstrated (Brandt, et al., 2009). The antispasmodic agents include those that directly affect intestinal smooth muscle relaxation (e.g., mebeverine and pinaverine), and those that act via their anticholinergic or antimuscarinic properties (e.g., dicyclomine and hyoscyamine) (Brandt, et al., 2009). The selective inhibition of gastrointestinal smooth muscle reduces stimulated colonic motor activity and may be beneficial in patients with postprandial abdominal pain, gas, bloating, and fecal urgency (Brandt, et al., 2009). Administration of these medications in the treatment of IBS should be on an as-required basis or prior to known stressors with predictable exacerbating effects.

Antidepressants — Antidepressants e.g. amitriptyline, Imipramine, nortriptyline, desipramine have analgesic properties independent of their mood improving effects and may therefore be beneficial in patients with neuropathic pain. The possible mechanisms of pain modulation with tricyclic antidepressants (TCAs) and possibly serotonin reuptake inhibitors (SSRIs) in IBS are facilitation of endogenous endorphin release, blockade of norepinephrine reuptake leading to enhancement of descending inhibitory pain pathways, and blockade of the pain neuromodulator, serotonin (Gorard, Libby, & Farthing, 1995). TCAs, have anti-cholinergic properties, therefore slow intestinal transit time, which may provide some benefit in diarrhea-predominant IBS (Clouse, Lustman, Geisman, & Alpers, 1994). Improvement in neuropathic pain with TCAs occurs at lower doses than required for treatment of depression. Because of the delayed onset of action, three - four weeks of therapy should be attempted before considering treatment insufficient and increasing the dose. The initial dose should be adjusted based upon tolerance and response. TCAs should be used cautiously in patients with constipation. Amitriptyline, nortriptyline, and imipramine can be started at a dose of 10 mg to 25 mg at bedtime and increased every three-four weeks based upon clinical response and tolerance.

Anti-diarrheal agents — In diarrhea-predominant IBS, the stools characteristically are loose and frequent but of normal total daily volume. A systematic review evaluated the efficacy of loperamide in the treatment of IBS (Brandt, et al., 2009). The three trials reviewed were of short duration, enrolled a small number of patients, and did not use standardized criteria for identifying patients. Overall, loperamide was more effective than placebo for treatment of diarrhea, but not for treatment of global IBS symptoms or abdominal pain. Administration on an as-required basis was preferred to a regular scheduled dosing in patients with diarrhea. Patients who consistently develop diarrhea after meals may benefit from taking a dose before meals, however, loperamide should not be used in patients with constipation and should be used only cautiously in those with symptoms alternating between diarrhea and constipation.

5-hydroxytryptamine (serotonin) 3 receptor antagonists— 5-hydroxytryptamine-3 receptor antagonists (such as alosetron, cilansetron, ondansetron and granisetron) regulate visceral afferent activity from the gastrointestinal tract and may improve abdominal pain (Andresen et al., 2008). A meta-analysis of 14 randomized controlled trials involving alosetron in IBS found a benefit in global improvement in IBS and relief of abdominal pain and discomfort (Andresen, et al., 2008). Alosetron was developed for use in IBS based upon its favourable effects on colonic motility, GI secretion and on the afferent neural systems. In clinical trials the drug was most effective in female patients in whom diarrhea was predominant. However, the drug was associated with ischemic colitis which has limited its use.

5-hydroxytryptamine (serotonin) 4 receptor agonists — Agonists of the 5-hydroxytryptamine-4 (5-HT4) receptor stimulate the release of neurotransmitters and increase colonic motility, thereby improving constipation-predominant IBS (Scott & Perry, 1999). The first of this class of drugs (Tegaserod, a partial 5-HT4 receptor agonist) was approved for IBS and constipation but removed from the market in March 2007 because of cardiovascular side-effects.

Lubiprostone — Lubiprostone is a locally acting chloride channel activator that enhances chloride-rich intestinal fluid secretion and can be used for the treatment of irritable bowel syndrome with constipation in women 18 years and older. There have been no comparisons with other options for treatment of IBS with constipation and its long-term safety remains to be established. At present it is best reserved for patients with IBS and severe constipation in whom other approaches have been unsuccessful.

Guanylate cyclase agonists — Linaclotide is a guanylate cyclase agonist that stimulates intestinal fluid secretion and transit and can be used for the treatment of IBS with constipation at a dose of 290 micrograms daily. However, the long-term risks of linaclotide are unknown and therefore its role on the treatment of IBS with constipation remains to be determined.

Antibiotics — Some patients with IBS have shown improvement when treated with antibiotics. Most of the improvement has been in symptoms of bloating, abdominal pain, or altered bowel habits. The randomized trials (TARGET 1 and TARGET 2) recruited 1260 patients with IBS but without constipation; rifaximin, a non-absorbable antibiotic when administered, led to symptomatic improvement in global IBS symptoms and bloating (Pimentel et al., 2011). The mechanisms leading to the benefit are unclear but may be due to suppression of gas-producing bacteria in the colon. Lactulose-breath testing for suspected bacterial overgrowth did not discriminate patients with IBS from healthy controls (Bratten, Spanier, & Jones, 2008) thus the relationships between bacterial overgrowth, its testing and benefits of antibiotics in patients with IBS require further study.

A review of clinical responses in KBTH, Accra

Table 13.5 illustrates the proportions of IBS and NUD patients on the respective therapies and their clinical response following 3 months of treatment. The available anti-spasmodics in Ghana include mebeverine 135mg and nospa-drotaverine 40 mg. Fifty percent (50%) of IBS patients on either anti-spasmodics (nospa-drotaverine 40 mg bid, mebeverine 135mg bid) or domperidone 10mg bid responded to therapy. Clinical response in IBS patients on amitryptyline 12.5mg nocte was seen in 35 percent of cases. (nospa-drotaverine 40mg bid-amitryptyline 12.5mg) combination therapy was however associated with symptom improvement in 61 percent of IBS cases. The use of *Helicobacter pylori* therapy in IBS was very low 4.3 percent with none responding to therapy. Patients with NUD exhibited a relatively poor response to PPIs (25.9 percent) despite a high prevalence of PPI use in this FBD group (79.1 percent). Clinical response was also low in NUD patients on Nospa-Drotaverine 40mg bid (25 percent) or following *H. pylori* therapy (25 percent) in comparison to domperidone 10mg bid or amitryptyline 12.5mg of use.

No pharmacological agent emerged superior in the management of FBDs. For instance, anti-spasmodics (nospa-drotaverine 40mg bid, mebeverine 135mg bid) or pro-kinetics (domperidone 10mg bad) were efficacious in 50 percent of IBS patients while clinical response in patients with NUD was seen in 43.5 percent on domperidone 10mg b.d and 25 percent on anti-spasmodics. There is current evidence supporting the benefit of antispasmodics in IBS (Ruepert et al. 2011) however domperidone therapy has revealed mixed responses with two trials showing no benefit and another demonstrating improvement.

There is limited efficacy of PPIs in FBDs as seen in our study population although PPI use was highly prevalent in NUD, 79.1 percent. The use of *helicobacter pylori* therapy was understandably low in the IBS patient-group and sustained clinical response following eradication therapy was poor in NUD. This would be in line with the lack of a definitive association between functional bowel disorders such as IBS and *H. pylori* infection. In reference to Table 13.5, amitryptylline 12.5mg had a relatively low response in IBS but this improved with (nospa-drotaverine 40mg-bid-amitryptyline 12.5mg) combination therapy to 61 percent.

The therapeutic responses in the NUD or IBS subgroups did not achieve statistical significance when compared with other FBD groups. This may be due to the relatively low sample size. Nevertheless, a significant placebo effect confounds the objective assessment of drug response in functional bowel disorders.

Limitations of this study include the possibility of bias in sampling or reporting in a retrospective records review. The study sample in a tertiary centre may also not reflect the situation in the community. It did not include the role of herbal or traditional agents in functional bowel diseases in Accra in a region where its use remains prevalent. It will, however, provide a basis for further investigation into illness behaviour and clinical epidemiology of functional bowel disease in Ghana.

Table 13.5: Irritable bowel syndrome and non-ulcer dyspepsia treatment response

Therapy	IBS patients (n=46)			NUD patients (n=43)		
	%(n) on therapy	Response (%)	P-value	%(n) on therapy	Response (%)	P-value
Nospa 40mg b.d	43.5% (20)	50.0	0.094	18.6% (8)	25.0	0.340
Mebeverine 135mg b.d	13.0 (6)	50.0	0.571	-	-	-
PPI once daily/ twice daily	34.8 (16)	37.5	0.306	79.1% (34)	25.9	0.383
Domperidone 20mg dly	26.1 (12)	50.0	0.208	53.5% (23)	43.5	0.237
H. Pylori eradication	4.3 (2)	-	0.662	37.3% (16)	25.0	0.249
Amitryjptyline 12.5mg dly	56.5 (26)	34.6	0.535	37.2% (16)	43.8	0.233

Conclusion

FBDs such as IBS and NUD are clearly multi-factorial in aetiology; therefore management relies on a holistic, bio-psycho-social, approach to care. Clinical presentation and the possible underlying patho-physiology of FBD guide the therapeutic trial: for instance, anti-spasmodics for colicky-(visceral)-pain syndromes, pro-kinetics for post-pyramidal dysmotility symptoms or TCAs e.g. Amytriptyline and selective-serotonin-re-uptake-inhibitors (SSRIs) for the modulation of visceral hypersensitivity. Non-pharmacological measures such as diet, lifestyle modification and psychological support play an important role in therapy as part of a multi-disciplinary approach to the care of the FBD patient.

References

Andresen, V., Montori, V. M., Keller, J., West, C. P., Layer, P., & Camilleri, M. (2008). Effects of 5-hydroxytryptamine (serotonin) type 3 antagonists on symptom relief and constipation in nonconstipated irritable bowel syndrome: a systematic review and meta-analysis of randomized controlled trials. *Clin Gastroenterol Hepatol, 6*(5), 545-555.

Bernersen, B., Johnsen, R., & Straume, B. (1996). Non-ulcer dyspepsia and peptic ulcer: the distribution in a population and their relation to risk factors. *Gut, 38*(6), 822-825.

Bijkerk, C. J., de Wit, N. J., Muris, J. W., Whorwell, P. J., Knottnerus, J. A., & Hoes, A. W. (2009). Soluble or insoluble fibre in irritable bowel syndrome in primary care? Randomised placebo controlled trial. *BMJ, 339*, b3154.

Bohmer, C. J., & Tuynman, H. A. (2001). The effect of a lactose-restricted diet in patients with a positive lactose tolerance test, earlier diagnosed as irritable bowel syndrome: a 5-year follow-up study. *Eur J Gastroenterol Hepatol, 13*(8), 941-944.

Brandt, L. J., Chey, W. D., Foxx-Orenstein, A. E., Schiller, L. R., Schoenfeld, P. S., Spiegel, B. M., et al. (2009). An evidence-based position statement on the management of irritable bowel syndrome. *Am J Gastroenterol, 104 Suppl 1*, S1-35.

Bratten, J. R., Spanier, J., & Jones, M. P. (2008). Lactulose breath testing does not discriminate patients with irritable bowel syndrome from healthy controls. *Am J Gastroenterol, 103*(4), 958-963.

Caldarella, M. P., Serra, J., Azpiroz, F., & Malagelada, J. R. (2002). Prokinetic effects in patients with intestinal gas retention. *Gastroenterology, 122*(7), 1748-1755.

Chang, L. (2004). Review article: epidemiology and quality of life in functional gastrointestinal disorders. *Aliment Pharmacol Ther, 20 Suppl 7*, 31-39.

Chey, W. Y., Jin, H. O., Lee, M. H., Sun, S. W., & Lee, K. Y. (2001). Colonic motility abnormality in patients with irritable bowel syndrome exhibiting abdominal pain and diarrhea. *Am J Gastroenterol, 96*(5), 1499-1506.

Choi, Y. K., Johlin, F. C., Jr., Summers, R. W., Jackson, M., & Rao, S. S. (2003). Fructose intolerance: an under-recognized problem. *Am J Gastroenterol, 98*(6), 1348-1353.

Clouse, R. E., Lustman, P. J., Geisman, R. A., & Alpers, D. H. (1994). Antidepressant therapy in 138 patients with irritable bowel syndrome: a five-year clinical experience. *Aliment Pharmacol Ther, 8*(4), 409-416.

Dobrek, L., & Thor, P. J. (2009). Pathophysiological concepts of functional dyspepsia and irritable bowel syndrome future pharmacotherapy. *Acta Pol Pharm, 66*(5), 447-460.

Dorn, S. D., Palsson, O. S., Thiwan, S. I., Kanazawa, M., Clark, W. C., van Tilburg, M. A., et al. (2007). Increased colonic pain sensitivity in irritable bowel syndrome is the result of an increased tendency to report pain rather than increased neurosensory sensitivity. *Gut, 56*(9), 1202-1209.

Drossman, D. A., Corazziari, E., Delvaux, M., Spiller, R., Talley, N. J., & Thompson, W. G.(2010) [Appendix B: Rome III diagnostic criteria for functional gastrointestinal disorders.]. *Rev Gastroenterol Mex, 75*(4), 511-516.

Drossman, D. A., Li, Z., Andruzzi, E., Temple, R. D., Talley, N. J., Thompson, W. G., et al. (1993). US. householder survey of functional gastrointestinal disorders. Prevalence, sociodemography, and health impact. *Dig Dis Sci, 38*(9), 1569-1580.

Gibson, P. R., & Shepherd, S. J. (2005). Personal view: food for thought--Western lifestyle and susceptibility to Crohn's disease. The FODMAP hypothesis. *Aliment Pharmacol Ther, 21*(12), 1399-1409.

Gonlachanvit, S., Fongkam, P., Wittayalertpanya, S., & Kullavanijaya, P. (2007). Red chili induces rectal hypersensitivity in healthy humans: possible role of 5HT-3 receptors on capsaicin-sensitive visceral nociceptive pathways. *Aliment Pharmacol Ther, 26*(4), 617-625.

Gorard, D. A., Libby, G. W., & Farthing, M. J. (1995). Effect of a tricyclic antidepressant on small intestinal motility in health and diarrhea-predominant irritable bowel syndrome. *Dig Dis Sci, 40*(1), 86-95.

Hirakawa, K., Adachi, K., Amano, K., Katsube, T., Ishihara, S., Fukuda, R., et al. (1999). Prevalence of non-ulcer dyspepsia in the Japanese population. *J Gastroenterol Hepatol, 14*(11), 1083-1087.

Kang, J. M., Kim, N., Lee, B. H., Park, H. K., Jo, H. J., Shin, C. M., et al. (2011). Risk factors for peptic ulcer bleeding in terms of Helicobacter pylori, NSAIDs, and antiplatelet agents. *Scand J Gastroenterol, 46*(11), 1295-1301.

Kassinen, A., Krogius-Kurikka, L., Makivuokko, H., Rinttila, T., Paulin, L., Corander, J., et al. (2007). The fecal microbiota of irritable bowel syndrome patients differs significantly from that of healthy subjects. *Gastroenterology, 133*(1), 24-33.

Keck, M. E., & Holsboer, F. (2001). Hyperactivity of CRH neuronal circuits as a target for therapeutic interventions in affective disorders. *Peptides, 22*(5), 835-844.

Kwan, A. C., Bao, T. N., Chakkaphak, S., Chang, F. Y., Ke, M. Y., Law, N. M., et al. (2003). Validation of Rome II criteria for functional gastrointestinal disorders by factor analysis of symptoms in Asian patient sample. *J Gastroenterol Hepatol, 18*(7), 796-802.

Ladep, N. G., Obindo, T. J., Audu, M. D., Okeke, E. N., & Malu, A. O. (2006). Depression in patients with irritable bowel syndrome in Jos, Nigeria. *World J Gastroenterol, 12*(48), 7844-7847.

Levy, R. L., Jones, K. R., Whitehead, W. E., Feld, S. I., Talley, N. J., & Corey, L. A. (2001). Irritable bowel syndrome in twins: heredity and social learning both contribute to etiology. *Gastroenterology, 121*(4), 799-804.

Locke, G. R., 3rd, Weaver, A. L., Melton, L. J., 3rd, & Talley, N. J. (2004). Psychosocial factors are linked to functional gastrointestinal disorders: a population based nested case-control study. *Am J Gastroenterol, 99*(2), 350-357.

Longstreth, G. F., Hawkey, C. J., Mayer, E. A., Jones, R. H., Naesdal, J., Wilson, I. K., et al. (2001). Characteristics of patients with irritable bowel syndrome recruited from three sources: implications for clinical trials. *Aliment Pharmacol Ther, 15*(7), 959-964.

Lule, G. N., & Amayo, E. O. (2002). Irritable bowel syndrome in Kenyans. *East Afr Med J, 79*(7), 360-363.

Mahadeva, S., & Goh, K. L. (2006). Epidemiology of functional dyspepsia: a global perspective. *World J Gastroenterol, 12*(17), 2661-2666.

Mahadeva, S., Yadav, H., Rampal, S., Everett, S. M., & Goh, K. L.(2010). Ethnic variation, epidemiological factors and quality of life impairment associated with dyspepsia in urban Malaysia. *Aliment Pharmacol Ther, 31*(10), 1141-1151.

Manning, A. P., Thompson, W. G., Heaton, K. W., & Morris, A. F. (1978). Towards positive diagnosis of the irritable bowel. *Br Med J, 2*(6138), 653-654.

Okeke, E. N., Ladep, N. G., Adah, S., Bupwatda, P. W., Agaba, E. I., & Malu, A. O. (2009). Prevalence of irritable bowel syndrome: a community survey in an African population. *Ann Afr Med, 8*(3), 177-180.

Pimentel, M., Lembo, A., Chey, W. D., Zakko, S., Ringel, Y., Yu, J., et al. (2011). Rifaximin therapy for patients with irritable bowel syndrome without constipation. *N Engl J Med, 364*(1), 22-32.

Ruepert, L., Quartero, A. O., de Wit, N. J., van der Heijden, G. J., Rubin, G., & Muris, J. W. (2011). Bulking agents, antispasmodics and antidepressants for the treatment of irritable bowel syndrome. *Cochrane Database Syst Rev*(8), CD003460.

Sainsbury, A., & Ford, A. C.(2011). Treatment of irritable bowel syndrome: beyond fiber and antispasmodic agents. *Therap Adv Gastroenterol, 4*(2), 115-127.

Scott, L. J., & Perry, C. M. (1999). Tegaserod. *Drugs, 58*(3), 491-496; discussion 497-498.

Shepherd, S. J., Parker, F. C., Muir, J. G., & Gibson, P. R. (2008). Dietary triggers of abdominal symptoms in patients with irritable bowel syndrome: randomized placebo-controlled evidence. *Clin Gastroenterol Hepatol, 6*(7), 765-771.

Solmaz, M., Kavuk, I., & Sayar, K. (2003). Psychological factors in the irritable bowel syndrome. *Eur J Med Res, 8*(12), 549-556.

Thabane, M., Kottachchi, D. T., & Marshall, J. K. (2007). Systematic review and meta-analysis: The incidence and prognosis of post-infectious irritable bowel syndrome. *Aliment Pharmacol Ther, 26*(4), 535-544.

Wahnschaffe, U., Schulzke, J. D., Zeitz, M., & Ullrich, R. (2007). Predictors of clinical response to gluten-free diet in patients diagnosed with diarrhea-predominant irritable bowel syndrome. *Clin Gastroenterol Hepatol, 5*(7), 844-850; quiz 769.

Zwetchkenbaum, J., & Burakoff, R. (1988). The irritable bowel syndrome and food hypersensitivity. *Ann Allergy, 61*(1), 47-49.

Chapter 14

Group Therapy for Mothers of Unwell Neonatal Infants

Hannah Belle A. Anang, Salma Yusuf Adusei, Ethel Akpene Atefoe, Yasmin Mohammed and Angela Ofori-Atta.

Introduction

Group therapy is a type of psychotherapy that involves one or more therapists working with several people at the same time. This type of therapy is widely available at a variety of locations, including private therapeutic practices, hospitals, mental health clinics and community centres. Group therapy is sometimes used alone, but it is commonly integrated into a comprehensive treatment plan that includes individual therapy and medication. Group therapy has been shown to be as effective as individual therapy for higher functioning adults (Gardenswartz, 2009).

People join therapy groups for different reasons. Some may be experiencing difficulties while others are looking for personal growth. Group therapy provides a unique way to learn about oneself and one's relationships and to give and receive support and feedback from others.

Having a baby can be one of the happiest and most important events in a woman's life. Despite the joy associated with the birth of a child, the period can also be very stressful for most mothers, especially if the baby is unwell. Inability to manage this stressful period properly could result in several consequences for both mother and child. About 80% of women experience mild mood disturbances following childbirth, often known as "baby blues" which usually resolves in a matter of days (Bennett & Indman, 2006). Between 7 and 26 percent often develop severe depression (postpartum depression) which requires clinical intervention (Robertson, Grace, Wallington & Stewart, 2004). Some may experience anxiety disorders such as panic disorder and obsessive compulsive disorder; characterized by obsession with the well-being of the child (Mehta & Sheth, 2006). According to Gjerdingen & Yawn (2007), postpartum depression is considered the leading psychological disorder in women after childbirth. They suggest that women who present with symptoms of postpartum depression usually remain at risk for depression throughout the postpartum year. Some of the risk factors for common postpartum disorders include; personal history of depression, limited social support, stressful life events, and lack of adaptive coping skills to deal with them, maternal personality (negative attribution styles, low self-esteem etc.), low socioeconomic status and obstetric complications (Robertson et al., 2004; Ryan et al., 2005).

In the Ghanaian culture, child birth is marked by several activities including a ceremony to announce the birth of the child and to honour the mother. Mothers are expected to adorn themselves in white clothes for a number of weeks, which makes them easily identifiable. Mostly, the woman's mother, mother-in-law or a family member goes to stay with her shortly after childbirth to help in taking care of the baby and the mother until she is strong enough to do that herself. This, we believe, in a way protects a new mother against postpartum depression and other psychological issues; lack of social support is, after all, one of the high risk factors for postpartum depression and anxiety disorders (Beck, 2001; O'Hara & Swain, 1996).

These Ghanaian practices, however, often do not apply to mothers whose newborns are unwell and are still in the Hospital (Neonatal Intensive-Care-Unit NICU). Most of these mothers are often culturally and physically separated from their support systems and their present experiences of motherhood differ significantly from their "cultural" expectations. Some of the mothers whose babies are brought to the NICU experienced obstetric and pregnancy complications which increase the likelihood of such mothers experiencing symptoms of depression and anxiety. It has been found that in Ghana, mothers who have sick babies are much more likely to suffer from postpartum depression (Gold, Spangenberg, Wobil & Schwenk, 2012). Thus,there is the need for these mothers to be given some form of social support while they are still in the hospital. Similarly, mothers who are at risk for postpartum depression and anxiety disorders should be identified and given the necessary help. These considerationss necessitated the introduction of some form of psychotherapy at the Neonatal Intensive Care Unit of the Korle Bu Teaching Hospital (KBTH). With the large patient: psychologist ratio, group therapy appeared to be the most feasible medium for this approah.

Related studies

Group therapy has been used in a number of studies on different populations; children, adults, and different clinical populations such as those involved in pathological gambling (Carlbring, Jonsson, Josephson, & Forsberg 2010) as well as depression (McDermut, Miller, & Brown, 2001) .

In relation to depression (which is the common presenting problem in our chosen population), group therapy has mostly been found to be effective. One of the landmark studies in this area was a meta-analytic review of one hundred and eleven (111) studies by Burlingame, Fuhman, & Mosier (2003), who reviewed studies published within a 20 year period and found an overall moderate effect size of 0.58. McDermut, Miller, & Brown (2001) provided a meta-analytic review of the effectiveness of group psychotherapy in the treatment of depression (for a review of their paper, see Truax, 2001). Of the 48 studies examined, 43 showed statistically significant reductions in depressive symptoms following group psychotherapy; nine showed no difference in effectiveness between group and individual therapy; and eight showed CBT to be more effective than psychodynamic group therapy. Cognitive–behavioural therapy (CBT) and psycho-educational cognitive therapy were originally prescribed for individuals and are now increasingly being provided to groups. There are now robust research findings showing the effectiveness of dynamic groups as a powerful intervention for a number of disorders, including depression, personality disorder and anxiety states (Robinson et al.1990; Budman et al., 1998).

Of the various approaches, cognitive therapy is the most practiced alternative (Hollon & Ponniah, 2010). Indeed, studies have reported cognitive therapy to be as effective as drugs and sometimes even more efficacious than drugs, especially with regard to the prevention of relapse.

Recently, more directed forms of therapy in relation to both the modality (individual or group) and type (cognitive, psychodynamic or otherwise) are being reported in the literature. For instance, a recent meta-analysis by Feng, Chu, Chen, Chang, and Chen, et al. (2012) was specifically on cognitive-behavioural group therapy for depression (CBGT). This study considered the total effectiveness of cognitive behavioural group therapy for depression with studies conducted between 2000 and 2010. With a total of 32 studies fitting their criteria, they found that CGBT had both an immediate and continuous effect for a period of 6 months after therapy. Even more importantly, , CBGT lowered the relapse rate of depression.

Why the choice of group therapy sessions with mothers at the Neonatal Intensive Care Unit (NICU), Korle Bu?

Psychotherapy groups may meet several times weekly. Opinions vary as to the appropriate goals and nature of such groups in this setting. Some theorists propose that it is the group itself that offers healing, and for others it is the individual interactions within the group. Kibel (1993) describes the overarching goal for an inpatient group as that of increasing the treatment alliance between staff and patients. He advocates inclusive group membership (excepting only the most disruptive or cognitively impaired patients) and a focus on helping patients improve relatedness, reality testing, and management of effect by helping them understand their experience in the milieu.

Group therapy in hospitals is more essential now than ever if patients are to feel a sense of purpose in regaining control of their lives and to rise above the sea of hopelessness that threatens inpatient care providers and their patients alike.

The therapy is centred around cognitive behaviour therapy (CBT) where the main assumption is that negative thoughts or distortions about events or experiences lead to changes in mood which are negative too. Thus, during two sessions, mothers are given a vignette describing a hypothetical situation similar to their own and asked what the hypothetical mother would think and how she would feel. They are then asked to say what they would think and how they would feel. As the group discusses these issues, therapists gently point out the link between thought and mood. In the second session, therapists describe a few common thought distortions (e.g. all or nothing thinking, heaven's reward fallacies, mind reading, etc.) and help mothers to challenge these distortions in the examples given by mothers themselves. Mothers are encouraged to participate in the two sessions before discharge, and to attend repetitions of the sessions if their babies remain longer so they can learn the cognitive skills better and also benefit from the bonds and warmth of the sessions.

As well, mothers are directed to focus on those issues that brought them into the hospital and are encouraged to help each other understand where their coping skills and defences break down. This is accomplished through a largely exclusive focus on events occurring within the group session.

The benefits of the group therapy sessions at NICU are worth noting. Since the therapeutic sessions began, most mothers have found them very helpful due to certain properties of the sessions similar to therapeutic factors suggested by Yalom and Leszcz, (2005). These include:

Acceptance and universalization: Most mothers reported that they had a feeling of being accepted by other members of the group (Yalom & Leszcz, 2005). The tolerance of differences of opinion also assured them of an absence of censure. Furthermore, the awareness that she was not alone in having problems, that others shared similar complaints and that she was not unique, gave mothers a sense of comfort. During the initial part of the sessions, where mothers introduce themselves to each other and told each other the reason for their baby's admission, they discovered that majority of babies were jaundiced, had acute respiratory distress, neonatal sepsis and were premature or underweight.

*Altruism:*The act of members being of help to one another; putting another person's need before one's own and learning that there is value in giving to others was a major factor in establishing group cohesion and community feeling (Yalom & Leszcz, 2005). Outside the therapeutic sessions, mothers were still able to comfort those who began to feel less hopeful when they found out that their babies' conditions had not improved or had worsened at the next feeding period or the following day at review.

Catharsis: Mothers reported that the expression of ideas, thoughts, and suppressed emotions was accompanied by an emotional response that produced a state of relief (Yalom & Leszcz, 2005). Very often in the middle of the sessions, some of the mothers would break down, express their anger or cry out their pain because it was the only safe place to express their emotions.

Cohesion: The sense that the group is working together toward a common goal, also referred to as a sense of we-ness engendered a feeling of belonging (Yalom & Leszcz, 2005). The goals for our therapy sessions were to provide support and to improve coping. Moreover, the free and open exchange of ideas and feelings among group members also engendered effective interaction even though the mothers were from diverse ethnicities and socioeconomic backgrounds. In fact, cohesion in the therapeutic relationship has been suggested to account for up to nine times greater impact on patient improvement than specific mechanisms in other treatment protocols (Wampold, 2001).

Contagion: This phenomenon is the process through which the expression of emotion by one member stimulates the awareness of a similar emotion in another member (Yalom & Leszcz, 2005). During some of the sessions, there were a number of mothers whose babies had been on the ward for some time, who made the more recent comers realize that they understood what they were experiencing at present and had also been at the same point a few days earlier and that their babies would get better in time.

Insight: This was achieved through conscious awareness and understanding of one's own symptoms of maladaptive patterns of thought (Yalom & Leszcz, 2005). The mothers were able to gain insight or awareness and understanding leading to positive changes in their emotions and behavior. The therapists were able to achieve this by the use of a metaphor; enabling the mothers to view their mind as a football pitch, the negative and positive thoughts that they choose to dwell on as the players and they themselves being the coaches that decide what thoughts are present on the field at a particular time and how these affect their emotions and behavior.

Inspiration: Most mothers also reported that the therapy sessions gave them a sense of optimism and the ability to recognize that one has the capacity to overcome problems, which is also known as instillation of hope. (Yalom & Leszcz, 2005). Usually, mothers would interpret their children being given oxygen or phototherapy as a worsening in the child's condition but other mothers whose babies had undergone the same procedures and had improved over time always reassured them that their babies would also improve in time.

Interpretation: The therapists believed that the way we interpret our situations affects the way we react to them so the therapists were able to explain the link between thinking, feeling and behavior (Yalom & Leszcz, 2005). The result was that the mothers were able to develop a cognitive framework within which to understand themselves.

Learning: Mothers also acquired knowledge about new areas, such as social skills and communicating; they received advice, obtained guidance, attempted to influence, and were influenced by other group members (Yalom & Leszcz, 2005). Mothers who had been at NICU for some weeks were able to teach the new mothers better ways to communicate and interact with the doctors and nurses so as to gain more information about their babies' condition and progress.

Setbacks

Despite the evidence and the positive attributes associated with group therapy, it is not a readily embraced form of treatment. An indication of this was reported by Budman et al. (1988), who conducted a study that compared time-limited group therapy and time-limited individual therapy for psychiatric outpatients. These investigators found significant improvement for patients in both types of treatment. However, they also found that patients tended to prefer individual therapy. Other formal and informal reports in the literature suggest that if they are given the choice, many patients and many therapists would choose individual therapy for the following reasons:

- It is difficult to overcome the natural resistance to speaking with strangers about one's intimate life. Problems of early shame and exposure account for many early group dropouts and are not conducive to trust building among the members.

- Therapists have observed a lack of regard for these boundaries from busy medical and nursing staff, who often interrupt groups to handle other matters with mothers during the group meeting.

When there is limited institutional support for groups on a unit, group leaders find themselves called upon to provide the maximum possible degree of stability and safety within whatever frame actually exists in the setting. Although attendance at groups may be a requirement for privileges in some units, participation in psychotherapy groups should be fully voluntary, and in some cases, it may best be considered a privilege in itself.

- A number of aspects of the group therapy situation can make it seem more intimidating and less appealing. Mothers often experience a sense of less *control* in a group versus individual therapy where many people influence the flow of events.

The sense of *individuality* may also diminish and the mother must accept that she is part of a group. There is also *the potential* for less complete *understanding* of the events that transpire in session. Group discussions often jump from topic to topic and from person to person. In addition, the mother may experience feelings that initially are difficult to understand.

- Groups also offer less *privacy;* mothers are continually exposed to other new mothers, and absolute confidentiality is impossible to guarantee.
- The sense of *safety* may diminish for many mothers in a group; this is related to less control but more explicitly to the fact that criticism can come from many directions from a number of people. Thus, issues related to perceived or actual loss of control, individuality, understanding, privacy, and safety often lead to greater apprehension and resistance about participating in group therapy relative to individual therapy. A case in point is when during one of the therapy sessions, one mother openly criticized another as not being strong enough for expressing her

pain and sense of hopelessness for the death of one of her twin baby boys that same morning.

- In addition, groups are more complicated to organize. An entire set of mothers must be assembled to begin at the same time. It may be difficult to obtain a sufficient number of referrals. If one or more patients back out, the coming together of the whole group can be delayed, and if the group loses members after it has already started, the life of the group can be threatened. There was an instance at NICU when one mother who had not found previous group therapy sessions helpful discouraged the other mothers from attending the session.

In busy teaching hospitals such as KBTH, there are few places one can find large, comfortable, quiet spaces for group therapy. Our sessions were held in the small visitors' room on the ward with no air conditioning and not enough chairs for all the mothers. Secondly, scheduling the right time for all mothers was difficult. Thirdly, it was difficult translating concepts from the English of CBT into Twi, the most widely spoken Ghanaian language, even for the native speakers of the language. Sometimes a third translation was needed for a mother who did not speak either and then a patient might offer to translate. Fourthly, occasionally, a mother with a dominant personality would take over the session and would ride roughshod over the emotions of a grieving mother and even though she would be checked in midstream, the harm would already have been done. Alertness of the therapist and quick and decisive intervention is required to forestall this and individual sessions needed for those mothers who bear the brunt of such unsupportiveness. Finally, it seemed like when the floodgates of emotions for mothers were released, they wanted to stay in the group and it was difficult for therapists to end the session.

Conclusion

Considerable evidence supports the efficacy, applicability, and efficiency of many forms of group therapy, especially in resource-limited settings such as ours. However, interesting and important research questions for us are whether adding group therapy to treatment for mothers at a teaching hospital actually serves a protective function against post- natal depression and psychosis, and to standardize the terms used in our local languages for depression, anxiety, psychotic thoughts, thought distortions etc. We hope that group therapy researchers will continue to mobilize the resources and energy that are required to conduct the studies that will increase our understanding of how and why group therapies are effective. Clearly this is what is needed to further advance knowledge in the field of group therapy.

References

Alonso, A., & Swiller, H. (1993). *Group therapy in clinical practice.* Washington, DC: American Psychiatric Press.

Beck, C. T. (2001). Predictors of postpartum depression: an update. *Nursing Research, 50,* 275-285.

Bennett, S. S. & Indman, P. (2006). Beyond the Blues: *A guide to Understanding and Treating Prenatal and Postpartum Depression.* USA: Moodswings press.

Budman, S. H., Demby, A., Redondo, J. P., *et al* (1998) Comparative outcome in time-limited individual and group psychotherapy. *International Journal of Group Psychotherapy*, 48, 38–63.

Budman, S. H., Demby, A., Redondo, J. P., Hannan, M., Feldstein,M., Ring, J., et al. (1988). Comparative outcome in time-limited individual and group psychotherapy. *International Journal of Group Psychotherapy, 38,* 63–86.

Burlingame G. M., Fuhriman A., & Mosier J. (2003). The Differential Effectiveness of Group Psychotherapy: A Meta-Analytic Perspective Group Dynamics: Theory, Research, and Practice Copyright 2003 by the Educational Publishing Foundation; 7(1), 3–12

Carlbring P., Jonsson J., Josephson H., & Forsberg L. (2010), Motivational Interviewing Versus Cognitive Behavioural Group Therapy in the Treatment of Problem and Pathological Gambling: A Randomized Controlled Trial. *Cognitive Behavioural Therapy*; 39(2): 92–103 doi: 10.1080/16506070903190245.

Feng C. Y., Chu H., Chen C. H., Chang Y. S., Chen T. H., Chou Y. H., Chang Y. C., Chou K. R. (2012). The effect of cognitive behavioural group therapy for depression: a meta-analysis 2000-2010. *Worldviews on*

Evidence-Based Nursing;9(1):2-17. doi: 10.1111/j.1741-6787.2011.00229.x. Epub 2011 Dec 16.

Gjerdingen, D. K. & Yawn, B. P. (2007). Postpartum depression, its relationship to maternal postpartum depression and implications for family health. Journal of Advanced Nursing, 45(1), 26-35.

Gold, K. J., Spangenberg, K., Wobil, P. & Schwenk, T.L. (2012). Depression and risk factors for depression among mothers of sick infants in Kumasi, Ghana. *International Journal of Gynecology and Obstetrics, in press.*

Hollon S. D. & Ponniah K. (2010). A review of empirically supported psychological therapies for mood disorders in adults. *Depress Anxiety*; *27(10)*: 891–932.doi: 10.1002/da.20*International Review of Psychiatry, 8,* 37-54.

Kibel, H. (1993). Inpatient group psychotherapy. In A. Alonso &H. Swiller (Eds.), *Group therapy in clinical practice* (pp. 93–111). Washington, DC: American Psychiatric Press.

McDermut W., Miller I. W., Brown R. A. (2001). The efficacy of group psychotherapy for depression: a metaanalysis and review of the empirical research. *Clinical Psychology: Science and Practice ;8:98–116.*

Mehta, A. & Sheth, S. (2006). Postpartum Depression: "How to recognize and Treat This Common Condition". *Medscape Psychiatry and Mental Health,* 11(1), 1-8.

O'Hara, M. W. & Swain, A. M. (1996). Rates and risk of postpartum depression--a meta-analysis.

Robertson, E., Grace, S., Wallington, T. & Stewart, D.E. (2004). Antenatal risk factors for postpartum depression: A synthesis of recent literature. *General Hospital Psychiatry, 26*, 289-295.

Robinson, L. A., Berman, J. S. & Neimeyer, R. A. (1990) Psychotherapy for the treatment of depression: a comprehensive review of controlled outcome research. *Psychological Bulletin*, 108, 30–49.

Ryan, D., Millis, L. & Misri, N. (2005). Depression during pregnancy. *Canadian Family Physician,* 51(8), 1087-1093.

Truax, P. (2001) Review: group psychotherapy is effective for depression. *Evidence-Based Mental Health*, 4, 82.

Wampold, B. (2001). *The Great Psychotherapy Debate: Models, Methods, and Findings*. New Jersey: Lawrence Erlbaum Associates.

Weiner, J. B., Widiger, T. A., Stricker, J. (2003). *Handbook f Psychology (Volume 8, Clinical Psychology)*. Hoboken: John Wiley & Sons.

Yalom, I. D. (1983). *Inpatient group psychotherapy.* New York: Basic Books.

Yalom, I. & Leszcz, M. (2005). *The Theory and Practice of Group Psychotherapy* (5th ed.). New York: Basic Books.

Yalom, I. D., & Lieberman, M. A. (1971). A study of encounter group casualties. *Archives of General Psychiatry, 25,* 16–30.

Chapter 15

Play Therapy; a Pilot Project Supporting Children Undergoing Cancer Treatment at the Korle-Bu Teaching Hospital

J. Osae-Larbi, R. Acquaah-Arhin, S. Mork, and A. Ofori-Atta

Introduction

Children with cancer face pain, fear, anxiety and depression, among other difficulties as they undergo diagnostic and therapeutic procedures (e.g. bone-marrow aspirations, surgical operations, infusion treatments) and deal with the side-effects of treatment including nausea, and weakness (Young, 2005). According to the World Health Organisation (WHO, 1998) almost all children with cancer experience pain at some point during their illness; pain caused by the cancer itself, by treatments, and by invasive diagnostic or therapeutic procedures, as well as incidental pain from related causes. A study conducted to investigate how the experience of pain varied during cancer treatment revealed that while procedural pain gradually decreased, treatment-related pain was constant and dominating (Ljungman, Gordh, Sorensen & Krueger, 2000). Wachtel, Rodrigue, Geffken, Graham-Pole, and Turner (1994) found that children awaiting invasive medical procedures have significantly higher state and trait anxiety. Results of a study which investigated the incidence and severity of post-traumatic stress disorder (PTSD) in childhood cancer indicated that a full constellation of PTSD symptoms could occur in children over the course of cancer treatment (Butler, Rizzi, & Handwerger, 1996).

A number of studies have proposed interventions to help children cope with distress during cancer treatment. These include information, modeling, music therapy, art therapy and cognitive behavioral therapy. According to Powers (1999), cognitive behavioral therapy has been demonstrated to be an empirically supported treatment for pediatric procedural pain. Coping skills training based on cognitive behavioral principles has been most widely used and evaluated. The critical components of coping skills training typically include breathing exercises, distraction techniques, visual imagery, and muscle relaxation (Zelikovsky, Rodrigue, Gidycz, et al., 2000). A study on the effects of distraction on fear, pain and distress during port access and venipuncture concluded that distraction has the potential to reduce fear and distress during port access and venipuncture (Windich-Biermeier, Sjoberg, Dale, et al., 2007).

Hypnosis is another intervention for pain management which employs relaxation techniques and mental imagery to produce changes in pain level. For children in chronic pain, these techniques are learnt and used to enter an altered state of mind. Whilst in this state, the therapist makes suggestions (e.g. to recall times of feeling happy and well) aimed at producing the desired changes in pain intensity (Kohen, 1991; Smith & Womack, 1987). Paediatric hypnosis has been shown to be effective in controlling chronic pain, and treatment and procedural discomfort in children with cancer (Lorenz et al, 2008). However, using hypnosis in a clinical setting is time consuming as teaching of techniques is usually tailored to individual developmental and learning needs.

Play therapy, a technique whereby the child's natural means of expression, namely play, is used as a therapeutic method to assist him/her in coping with emotional distress or trauma has also been established as a highly effective intervention (Play Therapy UK, 2011). For decades, children have been known to express their feelings, experiences and ideas through action – play, (Lebo, 1955). Play therapy employs a variety of techniques, using a play therapy tool kit to assist children to express themselves. Techniques include creative visualization, therapeutic storytelling, drama-role play, art-drawing, music, dance and movement, use of sand trays and the use of toys. In a clinical setting, play sessions may be tailored to children or offered in groups. Group approaches allow for information and knowledge sharing. They are effective in reducing physical symptoms and increasing adaptation; reducing social isolation and increasing social support (Curle, Bradford, Thompson, et al., 2005).

Objective: The purpose of this study was to provide children with relief from boredom and from pain as they underwent cancer treatment.

Method

Participants: Following approval of the project, children with the diagnosis of a malignant disease and either on admission on the main cancer wards of the Department of Child Health of the Korle Bu Teaching Hospital or accommodated at the mothers' hostel participated in play activities. Children on the ward were identified from the diagnoses in their hospital folders. At the mothers' hostel, rooms allocated to cancer patients were identified from the reception and a follow up was done. Once the children were identified we sought the permission of the parent or guardian to spend some time with the children.

Equipment: A laptop was used to show movies. Crayons, colour pencils and A4 sheets were used in drawing and colouring activities. Other tools used were story books, puzzles, animal and flower stickers, noise-making toys, dolls, and action figures.

Activities: Between January and June 2010, children residing in the mothers' hostel and those admitted on the wards were engaged in play activities on Mondays and Thursdays respectively. Play at both sites usually began between the hours of 12:00 noon and 2:30pm. At the hostel, the chief nursing officer's room was used for all activities while the classroom on the ward was used mainly for showing videos. Activities engaged in depended on children's age, wishes or interest, and strength at the time of play. Children from the age of 3, who were strong enough to sit up or move around, took part in picture drawing, colouring and pasting of stickers to decorate their beds. Activities included board and card games. Games that involved clapping, counting and singing were played with children. There was a movie time, where animated movies were mostly shown. Children were engaged in conversation whilst they played. For older children, conversations were directed to gain insights into their knowledge of cancer, the treatment they were receiving, what it meant to them, and how they felt about their experiences.

Children below the age of 2 and bedridden children mostly did not take part in the above activities as they were too weak to play or would not join the others. For such children, noise-making or light-generating toys were given to them for play. Stickers mostly chosen by their mothers were also pasted on their cups or bedside cabinets to cheer them up.

Measures: The Activity Participation Scale (APS), a single-item scale developed by the research team, was used to assess the level of participation and interest of each child involved in the play activities. The response categories of the scale were: 1= Not at all active, 2 = Barely active, 3 = averagely active, 4 = Active, 5 = Very active.

Main findings

Thirty children (20 males and 10 females) aged between 2 years six months and 12 years took part in the project. About half of the children were between the ages of two and five years. Many had not started school at the onset of the illness or had just begun pre-school. There were a few foreign nationals, mainly from Togo. There were 22 mothers as primary caregivers, two grandmothers, a father, an uncle and a family friend. Three children had their mothers and another relative as caregivers. Over 20% of the children on the wards were bedridden during play times due to feelings of weakness, critical stage of their illness or being on infusions. Those at the mothers' hostel were more active and mobile, and less dependent on their caregivers. The types of cancers encountered included Burkitt's lymphoma, Hodgkin's lymphoma, melanoma blastoma, leukemia, retinoblastoma, neuroblastoma, and cervical lymphadenopathy.

Observations and scoring of interest in activities was done during each play session and scoring was done jointly by team members. There was an initial mixed response, with some children being very interested in playing and others being unresponsive. Over time, majority of children (especially those with longer or frequent hospital stays) expressed interest in the activities. Bed-ridden children and others on the ward, as expected, mostly scored lower (1-3) on the APS compared to children at the hostel who mostly scored higher (3-5). It was observed that children were happy at the time of play when age appropriate and sensory-stimulating tools were used.

The effect of play techniques on procedural and treatment-related pain was observed in one child. Colourful stickers were used to distract the child who initially expressed intense pain by crying while undergoing infusion treatment. The child was asked to go through various colourful stickers of animals and other objects, and to choose his favourite ones. By doing that, the child was distracted from the pain and ceased crying. The main issue that came up during conversations with children was the pain they experienced as a result of their treatments.

Discussion

The project was aimed at relieving paediatric cancer patients of boredom (since they were mainly out of school and away from home) by offering new experiences to the usual clinical routines. The project also aimed to relieve children of treatment-related pain using distractive play tools. The children's age ranged from 2 years 6 months to 12 years, consistent with previous literature which reported that cancer is more frequently diagnosed among preschoolers and adolescents (Eiser & Jenney, 1996).

Ratings of children's level of participation during sessions indicated a good interest in the project. The majority of caregivers expressed interest in the project and confirmed its necessity, and looked forward to the weekly sessions. It was obvious that there were no such activities available to children while in hospital. The televisions on the ward and hostel for instance, were most often tuned to adult channels.

During play, older children usually talked about their families, friends, incidents that had occurred at home and their expectations of going back home. Those who had started school shared experiences from school and sometimes did paintings or played games relating to school work. Activities children engaged in most included drawing, colouring, making posters, solving puzzles and reading story books with pictures. When asked to make posters to be pasted around their beds, children mostly wrote about God and the fact that He loves them and would heal their disease. In relation to their illness, it was observed that a majority of older children had no idea about the nature, causes, and timeline of their illness. Only a few children knew their treatment schedule or timeline. However, almost all children reported pain, and delay in starting or absence from school as a consequence of their illness.

The successful reduction in pain using colourful stickers in the case of the child who was undergoing infusion treatment indicates that play therapy has the potential to distract children's attention from procedural and treatment-related pain. As explained by the gate control theory of pain (Melzack & Wall, 1982), a shift of attention from sensations of pain reduces pain perception. The case of this child, however, revealed that medically, not much is done to control pain during procedures as the child received no pharmacologic management for his pain.

Conversations with caregivers indicated that most of them had no idea what was wrong with their children. They had no basic information about the diagnosis, treatment options, treatment procedures and sometimes the side effects of those treatments. Caregivers were mostly too shy or afraid to talk to doctors. Differences in dialects and inability to speak and understand English meant some caregivers relied on other staff or caregivers to communicate with doctors. In addition, they demonstrated little knowledge about the psychological effects that cancer and its treatments can have on children and how this can be managed. The majority also showed very poor knowledge of the nutritional needs of children with cancer as most continued to feed their children on more starchy foods and fewer greens. Furthermore, there were expressions of concern about delays in getting test results from laboratories. Almost all caregivers admitted financial constraints and how often this interfered with their compliance with their children's treatment regime.

Implications for expansion of the programme

To expand the service, a complete play therapy tool kit is needed to involve children of all ages and at different stages of treatment. A sand box in the mothers' hostel (placed in the court yard) would give the ambulatory younger children on the ward the chance of going out of the ward and being around children of their age group. As reported by Curle et al. (2005), this may reduce social isolation and increase social support. The bed-ridden ones could be engaged more effectively with distracters like talking bears, party blowers, and virtual reality glasses. For older children, videos of others sharing their experiences of cancer— pain, treatment side effects, and being out of school— and how they coped might be very helpful. Considering the ages of the children in the play group, colourful walls might make the wards and hostel a bit "warm" and might help improve children's mood.

There is an urgent need for a dedicated room where children can play safely at anytime of the day and feel confident to express themselves. Sharing an office with the chief nursing officer at the hostel and a consulting room on the ward meant some sessions were cancelled or interrupted. Expanding the service would also require more volunteers and perhaps an increase in the allocated play times to allow for personalized activities for children at greater risk of psychological problems. Professional play therapists to train volunteers and guide children through evidence-based coping strategies are also needed urgently. Parents need training to effectively monitor, manage and support children's psychological wellbeing. The APS should be validated to accurately assess interest of this population in play activities. The Child-Adult Medical Procedures Interaction Scale-Revised (CAMPIS-R) (Ronald et al., 1997) and the FACES scale (Whaley and Wong, 1987) could be used to measure children's pain and other psychological outcomes. Finally, financial support will be fundamental to expanding such a service. Suggestions have been made to solicit the help of corporate bodies as part of their corporate social responsibility.

Challenges included; language barrier where children and their caregivers did not speak English and none of the play team members could communicate in their spoken local language. Starting conversations and carrying out activities such as storytelling and role-play was therefore a big challenge. Currently, the Oncology Unit of the Department of Child Health lacks an accurate database system as well as a mainstream psychological service to ensure that each child diagnosed with a malignant disease is identified and given appropriate psychological support. Involving newly diagnosed children and effectively tracking the progress of participants was therefore a major problem the project faced. Engaging the bed-ridden children in fun activities was also a great challenge in light of our limited play instruments. There were issues of acceptance by some medical staff and caregivers who did not regard this form of psychological support as an essential part of the treatment process.

Conclusion

Play techniques seemed to be associated with positive experiences of children receiving cancer treatment at the Korle-Bu Teaching Hospital. If well structured and implemented, this service could go a long way to make children's hospital stay much less boring and less painful. Standardization of appropriate evaluation methods is needed to objectively highlight the effects of an expanded version of the programme. To successfully involve all eligible children, future expansion of the programme should also include updating the database on children receiving treatment for cancer at the Korle Bu Teaching Hospital. The result of the study also encourages future research to focus on effective ways of bridging the language and communication barrier between children, caregivers and providers of play activities.

Acknowledgement

We thank Dr. Lorna Renner, Department of Child Health, UGMS, Anne Mensah Kufuor and Olive Okraku, Department of Psychiatry, UGMS for facilitating the project.

References

Butler, R.W., Rizzi, L. P., & Handwerger B. A. (1996). The assessment of posttraumatic stress disorder in pediatric cancer patients and survivors. *Journal of Pediatric Psychology,* 21, (4), 499-504.

Curle, C., Bradford, J., Thompson, J., & Cawthron, P. (2005). Users' views of a group therapy intervention for chronically ill or disabled children and their parents: towards a meaningful assessment of therapeutic effectiveness. *Clinical Child Psychology and Psychiatry,* 10, 509-527.

Eiser, C., & Jenney, M. (2007). Measuring quality of life. *Archives of Disease in Childhood,* 92, 348-350.

Kohen, D. P (1991). Applications of relaxation and mental imagery (self-hypnosis) for habit problems. *Paediatric Annals*, 20, 136-144.

Lebo, D. (1955). The expressive value of toys recommended for nondirective play therapy. *Journal of Clinical Psychology,* 11, 144-148.

Ljungman, G., Gordh, T., Sorensen, S., & Kreuger, A. (2000). Pain variations during cancer treatment in children: a descriptive survey. *Paediatric Haematology and Oncology,* 3, 195-197.

Lorenz, C., Yousif, N., & Boyse, K. (2008). Pediatric hypnotherapy: hypnosis helping kids. Available: http://www.med.umich.edu [February 2, 2010].

Melzac, R., & Wall, P. D., (1982). *The challenge of pain*. New York: Basic Books Mosby.Windich-Biermeier, A., Sjoberg, I., Dale, J. C., Eshelman, D., & Guzzetta, C. E. (2007). Effects of distraction on pain, fear, and distress during venous port access and venipuncture in children and adolescents with cancer. *Journal of Pediatric Oncology Nursing*, 24, 8-19.

Play Therapy UK. (2011). An effective way of alleviating children's emotional, behaviour and mental health problems - the latest research. Available at: http://www.playtherapy.org.uk [March 1, 2010].

Powers, S. W. (1999). Empirically supported treatments in pediatric psychology: Procedural-related pain. *Journal of pediatric psychology*, 24, 131-145.

Ronald, L. B., Lindsey, L. C., & Natalie, C. F. (1997). The child-adult medical procedures interaction scale-revised. *Journal of Pediatric Psychology, 22, 73-88.*

Smith, M. S. & Womack, W. M. (1987). Stress management techniques in childhood and adolescence. *Clinical Pediatrics*, 26, 581-585.

Wachtel, J., Rodrigue, J. R., Geffken, G. R., Graham-Pole, J., & Turner, C. (1994). Children awaiting invasive medical procedures: Do children and their mothers agree on child's level of anxiety? *Journal of Paediatric Psychology*, 19, 723-735.

Whaley, L. & Wong, D. L. (1987). *Nursing care of infants and children, 3rd ed.* St Louis: CV

World Health Organization (1998). Cancer pain relief and palliative care in children. Available at: http://www.stoppain.org [March 1, 2010].

Zelikovsky, N., Rodrigue, J. R., Gidycz, C. A., & Davis, M. A. (2000). Cognitive behavioral and behavioral interventions help young children cope during a voiding cystourethrogram. *Journal of pediatric Psychology*, 25, 535-545.

Chapter 16

Breaking Bad News

Seth Asafo

Introduction

I once witnessed a breaking bad news session at one of the departments in Korle Bu. A woman who lost her child was invited to the matron's room and told point blank "your child is dead" she broke down into tears wailing. As if that was not enough, they ushered her out of the office while she was still crying and two nurses followed her in harsh voices saying "don't cry, you can still have another one." Just then I saw another mother rush to her and say, "Yes", what they are saying is true. After all, your eggs are still there. You will have another." I was surprised at how short a time it took our healthcare providers to break such news and why it was done so bluntly. They provided no outlet for this mother to come to terms with her loss. There was no avenue for consoling this mother as well. For the short while I have worked in the medical setting, I have realised that the manner in which some healthcare providers communicate bad news is unprofessional. I have observed it is done without adequate preparation (standing in the ward or on corridors), intrusions are not checked, it is done bluntly and does not allow any time for healthcare providers to respond to patients emotions.

Breaking bad news is one of a physician's most difficult duties (Nordstrom, Fjellamn-Wiklund, & Crysell, 2011); yet medical education typically offers little formal preparation for this daunting task. There are varying definitions of bad news however. Buckman (1984) defines bad news as "any news that drastically and negatively alters the patient's view of his or her future". Bad news is always, in the "eye of the beholder," such that one cannot estimate the impact of the bad news until one has first determined the recipient's expectations or understanding. For example, a patient who is told that her back pain is caused by a recurrence of her breast cancer when she was expecting to be told it was a muscle strain is likely to feel shocked.

Breaking bad news can be particularly stressful when the clinician is inexperienced, the patient is young, or there are limited prospects for successful treatment (Shun, Dunn & Enrich, 2012; Ptacek &, Eberhardt, 1996). Anecdotal evidence in the Ghanaian medical setting seems to suggest that breaking bad news is somewhat restricted to news of chronic illness (AIDS, cancer and so forth), disability and death.

The process by which bad news is delivered not only affects the patient's comprehension of information (Maynard, 1996), but also may affect his/her satisfaction with medical care (Ford, Fallowfield & Lewis, 1996, 2010), level of hopefulness (Wouda & Vande Wiel, 2012; Sardell & Trierweiler, 1993), and subsequent psychological adjustment (Fallowfield, 2004: Slavin, O'Malley & Koocher, 1982). In view of the above, receiving unfavourable medical information may cause psychological harm (Pfeiffer, 1994).

Many patients desire accurate information to enable them to make important quality-of-life decisions (Ngo-Metzger, 2009). In spite of the rewarding benefit of being informed as a patient, others who find it too threatening may employ forms of denial, shunning or minimizing the significance of the information, while still participating in treatment.

Without proper training, physicians may tend to disengage from patients emotionally because of the discomfort and uncertainty associated with breaking bad news. Numerous studies show that patients generally desire frank and empathetic disclosure of a terminal diagnosis or other bad news (Ford, 2010).

Process of disclosure of bad news

The process of disclosing unfavourable clinical information to patients can be likened to other medical procedures that require the execution of a stepwise plan. Thus, the process of disclosing bad news can be viewed as an attempt to achieve four essential goals.

1. Gather information from the patient; this allows the physician to determine the patient's knowledge, expectations and readiness to hear the bad news;

2. Provide intelligible information in accordance with the patient's needs and desires;
3. Support the patient by employing skills to reduce the emotional impact and isolation experienced by the recipient of bad news;
4. Develop a strategy in the form of a treatment plan with the input and cooperation of the patient.

Although there are varying opinions about how to break bad news, there seems to be a lot of consistency with the six step SPIKES (Baile et al., 2000) model with each stage as a preparation for the next.

1. The first step is **setting up** the interview and it involves mentally rehearsing for the task ahead. This step includes reviewing the plan for telling the patient and how one will respond to the patient's emotional reactions or difficult questions. It is helpful to be reminded that, although bad news may be very sad for the patients, the information may be important in allowing them to plan for the future. Some basic guidelines for this step include familiarizing oneself with the case, physical arrangement of the place, arranging for some privacy: an enclosed room or if on the ward pull the curtains around you. Involve significant others with permission— this could include close friends or relatives of the patient's choice. Have both the patient and healthcare provider sit down as this will calm the patient and reassure him/her that you are not going to rush. Maintaining eye contact may be uncomfortable but it is an important way of establishing rapport. Avoid interruptions by putting phone on silent and locking the door (Minichiello, Ling, & Ucci, 2007).
2. The second step is assessing patients **perception.** This step involves assessing what the patient already knows about the condition. Before discussing the medical findings, the clinician uses open-ended questions to create a reasonably accurate picture of how the patient perceives the medical situation— what it is and whether it is serious or not. For example, "What have you been told about your medical situation so far?" or "What is your understanding of the reasons we did the MRI?"

Based on this information you can correct misinformation and tailor the bad news to what the patient understands. It can also accomplish the important task of determining if the patient is engaging in any variation of illness denial: wishful thinking, omission of essential but unfavourable medical details of the illness, or unrealistic expectations of treatment (Fallowfield & Jenkins, 2004; Lubinsky, 1999).

3. The third step is obtaining the patient's **invitation**; this step involves judging exactly how much a patient would like to know concerning diagnosis, prognosis and plan of treatment. While a majority of patients express a desire for full information about their diagnosis, prognosis, and details of their illness, some patients do not. Examples of questions asked the patient would be, "How would you like me to give the information about the test results? Would you like me to give you all the information or sketch out the results and spend more time discussing the treatment plan?" If patients do not want to know details, offer to answer any questions they may have in the future and ask for permission from them to talk to a close friend or relative concerning their diagnosis, prognosis and treatment plan
4. The fourth step is presenting the **knowledge**. This step involves the actual breaking of the news. Warning the patient that bad news is coming may lessen the shock that can follow the disclosure of bad news and may facilitate information processing (Greisinger, Lorimor & Aday 1999). Examples of phrases that can be used include, "Unfortunately I've got some bad news to tell you" or "I'm sorry to tell you that…" The one-way part of the physician-patient dialogue may be improved by a few simple guidelines. First, start at the level of comprehension and vocabulary of the patient. Second, avoid technical words and medical jargon words such as "spread" instead of "metastasized" and "sample of tissue" instead of "biopsy" are better choices. Thirdly, avoid excessive bluntness for example, "You have very bad cancer and unless you get treatment immediately you are going to die". Although you may

not want to give any false hope, there are other aspects of life a patient may lose interest in with such bluntness. Remember to give information in small chunks and check periodically as to the patient's understanding and when the prognosis is poor, avoid using phrases such as "There is nothing more we can do for you." Remember there is always something a health care provider can do such as providing comfort, pain relief, information, and other support (Minichiello, Ling, & Ucci, 2007)

5. The fifth step involves responding to patient's **emotions**; this is one of the most difficult challenges of breaking bad news. Patients and families respond to bad news in a variety of ways (Blume, 2009). Some respond emotionally with tears, anger, sadness, love, anxiety, relief, or other strong emotions (Lacquer, 2011). Others experience denial, blame, guilt, disbelief, fear, or a sense of loss or shame, or may even intellectualize why the situation is happening. A few may demonstrate reflexive psycho-physiologic responses such as "fight or flight or faint" reactions. Outbursts of strong emotions make many physicians uncomfortable (Ngo-Metzger, 2009; Slavin, O'Malley & Koocher, 1982). Give the patient and family time to react. Be prepared to support them through a broad range of reactions. For example, handing a patient a box of tissues as they cry only exemplifies the fact that it is normal for them to cry. Acknowledge patient emotions, ask them to clarify how they feel: "You appear to be angry. Can you tell me what you are feeling? Does this news frighten you? I imagine this is difficult news..." etc. In summary, observe the emotion (tearfulness, silence, shock), secondly, identify the emotion by naming it to oneself and clarify with the patient using open- ended questions; thirdly, identify the reason for the emotion – this is usually connected to the bad news but if you are unsure, clarify with the patient and finally, after allowing some time, let the patient know that you have connected the emotion with a reason.

6. The sixth step, involves **strategizing and summary**. This means establishing a plan for the next steps, including arranging for the appropriate referrals.(Baile et. al., 2000). Discuss potential sources of emotional and practical support, e.g., family, significant others, friends, social worker, psychologist, etc. Reassure the patient and family that they are not being abandoned and that the physician will be actively engaged in an on-going plan to help. Ensure patient will be safe when he or she leaves. Give contact information in case anything comes up.

Although the task of breaking bad news may be sensitive and complicated, proper training on how to go about it reduces stress for the doctor as well as the patient. For example, in a study by Shea in 2011, a major finding was that doctors who employed the SPIKES model in breaking bad news found it relatively easier to do it and their patients reported few depressive symptoms. The manner in which we break bad news affects the healthcare professional, the patients, public perception about the medical profession and our institutions as well.

When physicians are uncomfortable with giving bad news they may avoid discussing distressful information, such as a poor prognosis, or convey unwarranted optimism to the patient (Wouda & Vande wiel, 2012: Hudson et al., 2008; Maguire, 1985). Hence, there is the need for proper skills training in breaking bad news. Most medical undergraduate and postgraduate programs do not usually offer specific training in breaking bad news (Wouda & Vande Wiel, 2012;Tulsky et al., 1998) and most medical practitioners learn to break bad news by observing more experienced colleagues in clinical situations (Mayer, Cassel & Emmanuel, 1998). In a study by Baile et al. (1999; 2000) the SPIKES protocol was used in interactive workshops for oncologists and oncology fellows. As an outcome, before and after the workshop a paper and pencil test to measure physician confidence in carrying out the various skills associated with SPIKES was conducted. It was found that the SPIKES protocol in combination with experiential techniques such as role play can increase the confidence of faculty and fellows in applying the SPIKES protocol. Undergraduate teaching experience also showed that the protocol increased medical students' confidence in formulating a plan for breaking bad news (Maynard, 1998: Hobgood, Tamayo-Sarver, Hollar & Sawning, 2009).

It is therefore imperative that this skill be taught to medical students in the course of their training. Seminars as well as refresher courses on the subject must also be organised for medical practitioners (doctors, nurses, matrons etc.).

In conclusion, clinicians must be aware that the component of religion is another facet of our socialization that we need to be particular about with regards to breaking bad news and how patients accept or cope with such news. From personal observation, many patients use faith as a powerful barrier to being disturbed by bad news. In their opinion, showing weakness and breaking down is a sign of not having faith in God so until you probe further as a clinician, patients may not reveal their true emotions about bad news they have received.

References

Baile W & Buckman R. (2000). SPIKES - A Six Step Protocol for Delivering Bad News: Application to the Patient with Cancer. *The Oncologist* 5:302-311.

Baile W.F., Lenzi R., Kudelka, A.P. (1997). Improving Physician Patient Communication in Cancer Care: Outcome of a Workshop for Oncologists. *Journal Cancer Education*, *12*:166-173.

Buckman R. (1984) Breaking Bad News – Why is it so difficult? *British Medical Journal*, 288:1597-9.

Fallowfield L., Jenkins V. (2004). Communicating Sad, Bad, and Difficult News in Medicine. *Lancet Oncology*. 24; *363*(9405):312-9.

Ford S., Fallowfield L., Lewis S. (1996). Doctor-patient Interactions in Oncology. *Social Science and Medicine Journal*, *42*:1511-1519.

Greisinger A.J., Lorimor R.J., Aday L.A. (1997).Terminally ill cancer patients: Their most important concerns. *Cancer Practice Journal*, *5*:147-154

Hobgood, C. D., Tamayo-Sarver, J. H., Hollar D. W., Jr., Sawning, S. (2009). Grieving: death notification skills and applications for fourth-year medical students. *Teaching and Learning in Medicine, 21*, 207-19.

Hudson P., Quinn K., O'Hanlon B., Aranda S. (2008) Family meetings in palliative care: Multidisciplinary clinical practice guidelines. *Biomed Central Palliative Care* 2008, *7*:12

Lubinsky M.S. (1999) Bearing bad news: Dealing with the mimics of denial. *Genetic Counselling Journal, 3*:5 12.

Maguire P., (1985) Barriers to psychological care of the dying. *British Medical Journal, 291*:1711-1713.

Mayer R.J., Cassel C., Emmanuel E. (1998) Report of the task force on end of life issues. *American Society of Clinical Oncology*

Maynard D. W. (1996) On "realization" in everyday life: the forecasting of bad news as a social relation. *American Sociolology Review Journal, 61*:109-131.

Ngo-Metzger Q. (2009) Breaking bad news over the phone. *American Family Physician Journal, 1*:80(5)-520

Minichiello, T. A., Ling, D., & Ucci, D. K. (2007). Breaking Bad News: A Practical Approach for the Hospitalist. *Journal of Hospital Medicine,* 2(6): 415-421.

Nordstrom, A., Fjellamn-Wiklund, A., & Crysell, T. (2011). The effect of a role-playing exercise on clerkship students' views of death notification: the Swedish experience. *International Journal of Medical Education*, *2*:24-29.

Pfeiffer M.P., Sidorov J.E., Smith A.C. (1994). The discussion of end-of-life medical care by primary care patients and physicians. A multicentered study using structured qualitative interviews. *Journal of General Internal Medicine*, 9:82-88.

Ptacek J.T., Eberhardt T.L. (1996) Breaking bad news. A review of the literature. *Journal of the American Medical Association*, *276*:496-502.

Sardell A.N., Trierweiler S.J. Disclosing the cancer diagnosis. Procedures that influence patient hopefulness. Cancer 1993; 72:3355-3365

Slavin L.A, O'Malley J.E, Koocher G.P. (1982) Communication of the cancer diagnosis to paediatric patients: impact on longterm adjustment. *American Journal of Psychiatry,139*:179-183.

Shaw J., Dunn S., Heinrich P. (2012). Managing the delivery of bad news: An in-depth analysis of doctors' delivery style. *Journal of Medical Education Perspective*, *87*(2): 186-92.

Tulsky J.A, Fischer G.S., Rose M.R. (1998). Opening the black box: how do physicians communicate about advance directives *Annals of Internal Medicine,129*:441-449

Wouda J. C., Wiel H. B . van de (2012) The communication competency of medical students, residents and consultants. *Journal of Medical Education, 86*(1):57-62.

Section D
Research

Chapter 17

A qualitative study of stresses faced by Ghanaian medical students

Angela Ofori-Atta, Olive Okraku, Seraphim Mork, Abena Sarfo, E. Ghanney, A. Sefa- Dedeh and Sammy Ohene

Introduction

Medical students experience much stress throughout their period of study. The stressors include but are not limited to difficulties of clinical years, stressors associated with continuous assessments, economic constraints, relationship problems, personality problems, mental health problems, substance abuse training and inadequate social support (Sani M, Mahfouz MS, Bani I et al., 2012; Sreeramareddy, Shankar, Binu et al., 2007; Chandrashekhar, Sreeramareddy, Suri et al.,2010; Super, 1998). Although these stresses may be considered as part of the daily hassles which all students face, the stresses faced by medical students seem to be magnified by the large amount of academic workload they face, the limited amount of time they have and the excellence expected of them. The prevalence of depressive symptoms among medical students was 12.9%, significantly higher than in the general population according to a study conducted in Sweden by Dahlin, Joneborg & Runeson (2005), and in Saudi Arabia, the sense of belittlement felt by students from both students and peers contributed significantly to stress (Shoukat, Anis, Kella et al., 2010). According to a study conducted in Nigeria, medical students cited as stressors overcrowded accommodation, congested classrooms, prolonged and frequent strikes and lack of holidays (Omigbodun, Odukogbe, Omigbodun et al., 2006).

Gunderson (2001) quotes from a director of medical humanities and medical research at Dalhousie University in Halifax: "We want people who are driven, who are competitive, who can excel at everything that they do." This is a tall order indeed because this high expectation comes at a price; most medical students are so concerned with dealing with the workload at school that they forget to take care of their physical, emotional, social and spiritual needs and this leads them to experience stress. "Self-care is not a part of the physician's professional training and typically is low on a physician's list of priorities" according to Gunderson (also Tait, Shanafelt, Bradley, et al., 2002); Dyrbye, Thomas, and Massie (2008). In addition to neglecting their own health, Werner and Korsch (1976) report L.L. Stephen's words;

> *"the encounter with morbidity and mortality heightens the student's feelings of vulnerability. If he over-identifies with patients, he may suffer more and be unable to provide rational medical care. If he protects himself by dehumanizing patients, humane treatment suffers."*

Clearly, the medical student is caught between a rock and a hard place. In spite of this, a study from Norway concluded that the mental health of medical students in Norway did not differ significantly from that of the general public. However, the students recorded lower levels of general self-esteem than those of the general public. Additionally, male students reported less general self-esteem and more nervous symptoms than female students (Bramness, Fixdal, & Vaglum; 1991).

In Ghana, practical steps are yet to be taken to identify the stresses that are experienced by Ghanaian medical students and the methods that can be used to prevent and alleviate them in order to prevent students from dropping-out.

Participants and methods

Selection of participants

After seeking permission from the University's administration, the class lists for medical students in Level 200, Level 300, the first clinical year and second clinical year were obtained. Every tenth student on the class list was selected to ensure random sampling from each class, after which the class presidents were added. They then participated in focus group discussions.

Procedure

The selected students were invited to the Department of Psychiatry at a time that was convenient for both the students and the staff at the department. Before focus group discussions began, the students were informed of the aims of the focus group discussion and their consent was sought. The students were assured confidentiality. A facilitator initiated the discussions by posing open-ended questions inquiring about stressors typically faced by medical students. This led to further discussions on topics including academic workload, food, accommodation and hostel facilities, relationship problems, financial problems, entertainment, religion and social support. Participants proposed possible solutions. These discussions were recorded with student permission by a simple digital voice recorder.

Analysis of data

The recordings of the focus group discussions were transcribed and emerging common themes on various stresses were identified. Similarly, solutions suggested by participants were noted.

Results

Principal stressors universal to students at all levels

All the four classes interviewed identified three major stressors: academic workload, promotion to a higher educational level from a lower one and financial problems as the main sources of stress in their lives. Concerning the academic workload, one female student had this to say:

> *"Mine has to do with work load. You realize that when in a day you don't just have a lecture on one subject. You have about two/three in a day and each one of them come and you get a whole lot of pages in your notebook to revise when you go back. But you realize that because each one of them is a lot, you get back and you don't get time to revise them..."*

The same student suggested restructuring the curriculum in such a way that related topics were taught successively instead of in isolation.

With respect to the difficulties faced as one moved from a lower to higher academic level, not only did the increasing workload pose a problem but the commute from Legon to Korle Bu and back each day was also identified as a time consuming process. The two campuses are approximately an hour and a half's journey apart in the mornings, and two on the return trip.

An overarching concern of students was the financial burdens associated with medical school. One student expressed this by saying,

> *"Because it is surprising that you have to come here after paying those fees, we have fee paying Ghanaian students, you understand. After paying those huge sums of money we go for practicals and you have to buy your own stuff."*

To that concern, another student proposed that materials such as books and laboratory supplies be subsidized by the government.

Although several students find the cost of books and other laboratory equipment high, the pressure is worse if the student is classified as a fee-paying student. One female student explained this phenomenon by saying,

> *"A lot of people don't speak about it. It's about fee-paying students. Like when we get admitted to school, I figure out a lot of people that didn't make it to the interview that were fee paying actually accept it maybe because somebody's promised or hoping they will get help later and then when they come... when they come to the school then they stress. They become very stressed out because the fees aren't paid. The school is asking for them to pay. They are thinking about how to pay about GH¢3000 or GH¢2500 or GH¢700."*

Other Stressors Universal to Students at All Levels

Another prominent source of stress identified by the groups was the unavailability of affordable food. Those who chose to cook found that it was a time-consuming and costly activity as explained by one student –

> *"Now you have to use the money you can use for other things to buy food. And since you don't, I mean you don't have the time as well to cook, so you have to use the money you have to keep, I mean, for other things to buy food. That and you know that Korle-Bu is way, way more expensive than even Legon. So I mean within a day you can spend GH¢10 without knowing it, just on food. Not even maybe a book or something. Because you are buying GH¢3 lunch, I mean breakfast is around GH¢2."*

Poor and inadequate hostel facilities appeared to contribute to the stress of medical students at all stages of medical school. One male student addressed the specific housing problems:

> *"I don't know but it seems like we are actually kind of separated from the other hostels in terms of our electricity power and our water sources. Sometimes you realize that the other hostels may be having light and we may not be having light in our hostel. It causes so many problems: sometimes our refrigerators, our deep freezers, and our laptops... You know sometimes our food goes bad. And sometimes it takes for us having to go to another person's hostel."*

With regards to religion, the main concern of the students who identified it as a stressor was their inability to balance their religious activities with their academics. Balancing other priorities such as relationships and entertainment activities also seemed to contribute to the stress of the students and for several of these students, this inability to find a suitable balance was due to insufficient time on the hands of a typical medical school student. One male student stated:

> *"Most of our friends, those we left behind and those doing other courses, because of the stress we are having now, we can't call them, can't visit them like we used to do last year."*

The current **structure of the medical school** was a cause of stress for several of the medical students. According to one of the students, due to their large numbers, several medical students were required to examine a single patient causing that patient distress. Additionally, medical students rarely interacted with faculty outside the allocated class time.

Stressors specific to particular groups of students

Aside the afore-mentioned stresses, the Level 200 class also identified the temperature in the auditorium, the African Studies class and the lack of problem-based and research-oriented learning as part of the difficulties they faced.

A stressor peculiar to the Level 300 class was personal pressure. One male student indicated that for him, maintaining a high level of discipline is a personal challenge he faces as a medical student. The second clinical year students also identified stressors associated with leadership as a source of stress.

In the second clinical year class, some of the medical students identified their source of stress as being their own health issues. They complained that after reading about or coming in contact with patients with particular diseases they became fearful and believed that they contracted those diseases and this became a major source of stress for them.

Stressors specific to the gender of the students, such as anxiety of the female students about the appropriate time to start a family, were also identified. This is illustrated by the words of one female student:

> *"I'm turning 30 next year, you know. It's like when am I going to have my kids? ... Do I have them now? ... All these things are coming up now and I wouldn't have that issue if I was a man."*

The Ghanaian female students identified the menstrual cycles as a source of stress. Apart from the experience of pain, which affected their attention in class and their ability to study out of class, they also experienced moodiness that negatively affected their relationships with others. One female student illustrates this point by saying

> *"Even before the menses alone, it comes with so many symptoms... you feel like ignoring everything.... You can just forget about your books and then even when your friend calls you, you feel like giving it to her there and then. You just forget about everything. It makes you behave in a particular manner, which doesn't help you to really move on with what is going on. You get lost in the class at any time and it doesn't really help so when you come back you will be far behind. And I'm also the first born and a female for that matter, so anytime there is a problem at home, they have to call on me and if I have to go, maybe for a whole weekend. My dad will just, he is not feeling well so anytime he calls you, you have to be there. If you don't go, it will be like, oh, you people, you don't take good care of me and all that. So if I have an IA[1] to write on Monday, I just have to put everything aside and go to be with him because he is paying my school fees. I have to go and comfort him and a whole lot of things before I come and it's not easy. It's not easy."*

From this student's experience it appears that certain students endure the added stress of depending on others for financial support and/or the responsibility of caring for aging parents and family.

Coping strategies employed by medical students

Several of the medical students sought ways of coping with the stress they endured. According to one female student, her colleagues in higher levels motivated her:

> *"... and you see MB3[2] students, the way they dress, the way they are friendly. If this person can do it why am I stressing myself, so I can do it also."*

Others employ humor and laughter to cope with the difficulties they faced:

---

1 IA represents Interim Assignment

2 MB3 represents the 3rd year of the Bachelor of Medicine Degree.

> *"...The workload I think is drastic from biological science to medical school, and is a lot of stress, so sometimes what I do to free myself or get it off is to joke. By telling jokes I make myself happy."*

To some, spending time engaging in a relaxing activity eases the stress. A male student who utilizes this technique says,

> *"For me, I pile up stress from Monday to Friday. Friday evening I don't study, I pick up my guitar, visit my female friends, sit with them and try and sing and play...but the issue is when I come back and take my books I realize I have so much to learn, then the stress starts. "*

Religion serves as a coping mechanism for some of the medical students such as the male student who said,

> *"Sometimes I encourage myself with scriptures, as God saw me through Biological Science, through the interview and up to this time. I encourage myself that He will see me through."*

For several students, having a special person in whom they may confide allows them to deal with stress. A female student who employs this coping strategy says:

> *"For me, I'm someone who is strongly attached to my father, yeah, and anytime I'm stressed out, just a call from my father, talking to him on phone is ok to make me fine, but right now there is a special friend too who I always go to."*

Discussion

There have been several studies done worldwide on the stresses faced by medical students in terms of the causes of those stresses and possible solutions. However, no formal research has been conducted on Ghanaian medical students. This research shows that like other medical students around the world, Ghanaian students also face a significant level of stress. The four classes interviewed identified the large volume of academic work, financial concerns, increasing stress levels from a lower academic level to a higher level and the stress associated with a student's gender as their main sources of stress. In 2001, Levey noted that medical students are stressed by heavy workloads, relocation issues, financial concerns and many others (Levey 2001). The medical schools in Ghana exert these same pressures on their students. There is, therefore, a lot of pressure on the Ghanaian medical student to keep up with academic work. They experience much financial pressure since the cost of living on campus or in hostel facilities is higher than at home.

In a related study (Sreeramareddy et al., 2007) it was noted that as students move from a lower class to a higher class, their stress levels decreased. However among the Ghanaian medical students, the stress levels seem to increase from a lower educational level to a higher one. It is worth noting here that up until 2011, medical students in Ghana were required to complete the first and second years of their undergraduate education prior to applying to the actual School of Medicine and this may account for the higher level of stress associated with moving from a lower educational level to a higher one. This quotation from one of the students in his first year in medical school may well illuminate the above:

> *"Sometimes it's very difficult to learn what we have because now what we have is very voluminous as compared to Level 100. Because right now, the handouts we are having for one course, is even more than Biological Science the whole year, than what we had before..."*

Among Ghanaian medical students, the general consensus was that being female was a disadvantage. This is in line with a study by Clark and Rieker (1986) which reported on gender differences in terms of the source and degree of stress perceived by students (Firth, 1978). In Clark's study, women were shown to be significantly more stressed than men. Furthermore, the women found sexism and difficulties with partners to be particular sources of stress, unlike the men. Despite the fact that both men and women indicated that the stress of their professional training had resulted in strained personal relationships, more women than men stated that their personal relationships had ended.

The students complained that being female limited the extent of a person's extracurricular activities since the few entertainment activities such as gymnasiums and television rooms were used mostly by males. When opportunities arose during vacations to gain extra clinical experience in the hinterlands, the females complained that their gender prevented their families from allowing them to take advantage of such opportunities since their families were afraid that something bad would happen to them in such remote places. Their male counterparts, however, found it easy to take advantage of such opportunities. Another source of distress that the female medical students complained about was the age at which they would be able to start a family. The male medical students believed that they could start a family at anytime even in later life but the females believed that it would be more difficult for them to start a family especially in later life. They also believed starting a family now would increase their stress levels because they would have to play the additional roles of wife and mother, which is especially demanding in our Ghanaian setting. A few females and males felt that being female was an advantage and being male a disadvantage. They expressed the opinion that females received more attention and more academic help from their peers and other members of staff such as lecturers and laboratory assistants. There were some students who believed that their gender did not affect their level of stress. A quotation by a female student may well explain the above discussion:

> *"for me... there are positives and negatives. Like the teaching assistants, when you want to work on microscope and all those things.... Please I can't see this or I can't see the brachial plexus or whatever.... You can call and then if you want to meet a guy even though he does not know you, he'll try as much as possible to ... then it's negative in a way because we are girls and we are growing, you have menstrual cycle. As for me it's very painful and I still have to come to school with that so I am thinking of my tummy, you are thinking of what the lecturer is saying, in fact it's something. If it was Biological Science you can say you'd miss a class ...... here, you can't. I'm not in a relationship though I was. But I know what it takes, like there are some guys not like this friend anyway, they are very caring and then sometimes they come to your room*

> *almost every time. They want to spend time but they don't understand that you can't spend as much time as you were spending with this person like when you were in level 100; like you had enough time and when you say I want to study, it's like you are pushing him away; you don't like him anymore, someone else is coming in-between and then as a girl also when he starts liking other girls you become jealous putting stress on you. That kind of thing."*

Ultimately, female students appeared to be more stressed than male students due to factors associated with their gender.

Other prominent stressors identified were time, food, poor and inadequate hostel facilities, religion, relationships, organization of the hospital and entertainment activities. According to Chandrasekhar et al. (2007) the most common sources of stress experienced by students were related to academic and psychosocial concerns in Nepal. The most important and severe sources of stress were staying in the hostel, high parental expectations, vastness of syllabus, tests/exams, lack of time and facilities for entertainment. Ghanaian medical students faced similar problems. Some students complained that their families and peers expected them to perform as they did in their previous classes or levels. The lack of time and facilities for entertainment also contributed to the stress of the students.

Time is an important component of success in medical school. Time to study, time to cook and eat, time to interact with family and friends all count towards a balanced and a successful life in medical school. Unfortunately Ghanaian medical students complained that they did not have time to fulfil all the obligations expected of them and this resulted in them experiencing a significant stress.

The students also identified food as a source of stress. Good food on campus was thought to be expensive and not readily available. Students expressed fears about not being sure about whether the food they bought on campus was hygienic. For those who chose to cook, especially, among the female medical students, there were complaints about not having enough time to cook.

For Ghanaian medical students, religion was identified as both a source of stress and a coping mechanism. The issue of time arose again in relation to religion. The students complained that they did not have enough time to cater to their religious obligations. Their stress was not only from their inability to partake in their religious activities but also pressure from their friends who belong to the same religious groups about their failure to meet their religious obligations A female student expressed this by saying:

> *" For me I have church services like almost every day of the week apart from Tuesdays and Thursdays and on Tuesdays I still have African Studies so by the time we get back... we leave here around 5pm with the traffic and everything you get to school after 6. When you get back 6:30pm, you have to be in church and if you don't go it's like when in Level 100 biological science, you were able to because sometimes you don't have lectures every day then ... you have one lecture a day and on Fridays just once and so I was able to go to church and then if you don't go to church in Level 200, God has done something for you and you are not appreciative. You know people are bound to say different things so by the time you get back, go to church and you want to come back and read, it's not possible so you end up not reading that day apart from lectures you had that day."*

As a coping mechanism the students stated that whenever they felt overwhelmed by other stresses, they turned to religion to seek comfort as one male student explains:

> *"... I also find church activities especially services when you are really down, I mean extremely down, especially when it's as if you're at the crossroads... I feel very ok when I get to the church and pray and worship..."*

Another source of stress identified was relationship stress. According to Firth (1986), relationships with consultants raised the strongest negative feelings, with 102 (34 percent) students finding these particularly stressful in the UK. Ghanaian medical students felt that they did not have enough time to form new or maintain existing relationships.

This was a major source of stress to them since they felt bad about not being able to make new friends, communicate with their lecturers or keep up with old friends.

The organization of the teaching hospital and medical school appeared to pose a problem for several of the medical students enrolled in the study. The large number of students made examining patients a cumbersome task. One female student expounded on this by saying,

> *"...a stress that has been consistent throughout the years is our numbers. Because there are so many of us in one ward, the patients get tired when we have to go and examine them for our sake."*

With respect to the Medical School, students indicated that clashing exam timetables, lack of correspondence between classroom and practical work and the overall poor organization of the academic timetable were a great source of stress. A male student commented on the poor academic timetable structure by saying,

> *"Two or three IAs (interim assessments) are put on one day and that increases tension."*

Due to the large number of stressors specific to the structure of the Medical School, an interview was conducted with an official at the administration office. It appears that about once a year, a forum is held for the medical students and staff in order to facilitate the discussion of problems faced by the students and possible solutions. With respect to the food situation of students, apparently none of the public tertiary institutions make providing meals to students a priority. It is not a problem exclusive to medical students. However, in an attempt to alleviate this stress, the Medical School has supported the construction of a structure for food vendors. Additionally, a Dean's guesthouse and service canteen located on campus provide meals to all. This addresses the issue of food availability but since the price of the meals are not subsidized by the Medical School, students are still faced with the challenge of meeting the cost. With regard to the commute, Legon and Korle Bu, the system has existed for many years and is unlikely to change in the near future. The students, however, do not need to find their own means of transportation since the university provides buses. Lastly, according to the administration staff member interviewed, the seemingly large academic load of the students may be as a result of there being a larger number of holidays during the course of the medical course than was the case in the past. Support is provided to the students by means of academic emotional counselors as well as remedial classes and it is up to the student to take advantage of these resources.

Recommendations

From the focus group discussions, the following were deduced as possible solutions to reduce stresses experienced by medical students:

a. Providing a more structured, problem-based and research-oriented academic system; providing better financial aid packages; building more hostels, canteens, recreational centers for males and females as well as comfortable, friendly lecture halls.
b. Psychological services should be incorporated in the university's system so as to help ease the stress these students face.
c. The main crux of the issue when it comes to stress is the limited time and the voluminous workload the students have. The university should therefore incorporate classes in time management and discipline into the syllabus.
d. The medical students and staff alike ought to endeavor to be more proactive in implementing the solutions they come up with during Academic Day.
e. The medical students themselves could be taught to assume an internal locus of control whereby they try to find positive solutions to their problems rather than leaving it entirely up to the university authorities to alleviate their stress.

Conclusion

Ghanaian medical students face similar stressors as other medical students around the world. Currently, the practice of holding student/staff fora is an avenue for medical students to voice their problems and challenges in order to collaborate with faculty to find solutions. Long-term solutions to issues pertaining to housing, academic structure and food are best addressed by the administration whereas stresses due to the demands of life as a medical student require that the individual student learns self-management skills such as how to cope by either seeking support or identifying an outlet such as extracurricular activity, and perhaps the Medical School ought to look into the provision of infrastructure towards this. Further studies should be done on the relationship between ethnicity, socio-economic status, pre-existing medical conditions and the associated stress faced by medical students.

References

Bramness, J.G., Fixdal, T.C., Vaglum. Effect of medical school stress on the mental health of medical students in early and late clinical curriculum. *Acta Psychiatr Scand.* 1991 Oct;84(4):340-5.

Chandrashekhar, Sreeramareddy, Sushil et al., (2010). Self-reported tobacco smoking practices among medical students and their perceptions towards training about tobacco smoking in medical curricula: A cross-sectional, questionnaire survey in Malaysia, India, Pakistan, Nepal, and Bangladesh. Available at :http://www.substanceabusepolicy.com/content/5/1/29

Clark, E. J, Rieker P P. Gender differences in relationships and stress of medical and law students. *J Med Educ.* 1986 Jan;61(1):32-40.

Dahlin, M, Joneborg N, Runeson B. Stress and depression among medical students: a cross-sectional study. *Med Edu*c. 2005 Jun;39(6):594-604.

Dyrbye, L, Thomas M, Massie, S. et al. (2008) Burnout and Suicidal Ideation among U.S. Medical Students. *Annals of Internal Medicine.* 149(5):334-341.

Firth, J. (1986). Levels and sources of stress in medical students. *British Medical Journal,* 292, 1177 – 1180.

Gundersen L. Physicians Burnout. *Annals of Internal Medicine.* 2001 Jul; 135(2):145-148.

Levey, R. E.(2001). Sources of Stress for Residents and Recommendations for Programs to Assist *Them. Acad. Med.* ;76:142-150.

Omigbodun, O.O., Odukogbe, A.T.A. Omigbodun, A.O., et al.(2006). Stressors and Psychological Symptoms in Students of Medicine and Allied Health Professions in Nigeria. *Social Psychiatry and Psychiatric Epidemiology.* 41 (5): 415 – 421.

Shanafelt, D., Bradley, K., Wipf, J., Back, A (2002). Burnout and Self-Reported Patient Care in an Internal Medicine Residency Program. *Annals of Internal Medicine.* Mar;136(5):358-367.

Shoukat, S., Anis, M., Kella, D. K., Qazi, F., Samad, F., et al. (2010) Prevalence of Mistreatment or Belittlement among Medical Students – A Cross Sectional Survey at a Private Medical School in Karachi, Pakistan. PLoS ONE 5(10): e13429. doi:10.1371/journal.pone.0013429

Sreeramareddy, C., Shankar, P., Binu, V. S., et al.(2007). Psychological morbidity, sources of stress and coping strategies among undergraduate medical students of Nepal. *BMC Medical Education* .7:26.

Sani, M., Mahfouz, M.S., , Bani, I., et al. (2012). Prevalence of stress among medical students in Jizan University, Kingdom of Saudi Arabia. *Gulf Medical Journal.* 1(1): 19 – 25.

Supe, A.N (1998) A study of stress in medical students at Seth G.S. Medical College. *J Postgrad Med*; 44:1-6

Werner, E. R., Korsch B.M. The Vulnerability of the Medical Student: Posthumous Presentation of L. L. Stephens' Ideas. *Official Journal of the American Academy of Pediatrics*, 57, (3), 321 – 328.

Chapter 18
Is the Concept of Learning Disabilities Applicable to Ghana?

Dzifa Attah and C. Charles Mate-Kole

Introduction

By far the most commonly noted characteristic of students with learning disabilities (LD) is their struggle with school work (Friend, 2008). At a general level, learning disabilities are first noticed when a child fails to learn academic material and requires school-based remediation to improve functioning (Cowardin, 1998). A student with LD possesses the requisite potential for particular academic activities, but has difficulty acquiring associated academic skills (Tanner, 2001). The LD tends to affect how much the student takes in, retains, or expresses information, hence impeding the child's ability to learn to read, write or do math (Mash & Wolfe, 2007).

Since the inception of research on learning disabilities (LD), several definitions have been used (Interagency Committee on Learning Disabilities, 1987; National Joint Committee on Learning Disabilities, 1998) to conceptualize LD. One commonly reviewed definition is that postulated by the National Joint Committee on Learning Disabilities (NJCLD, 1998). The NJCLD defined learning disabilities as a generic term referring to a heterogeneous group of disorders manifested by significant difficulties in the acquisition and use of listening, speaking, reading, writing, reasoning, or mathematical abilities. These disorders are intrinsic to the individual, presumed to be due to central nervous system dysfunction, and may occur across one's life span. Problems of self-regulatory behaviour, social perception, and social interaction may exist with learning disabilities but do not by themselves constitute a learning disability. Although learning disabilities may occur concomitantly with other handicapping conditions (for example, sensory impairment, mental retardation, serious emotional disturbance), or with extrinsic influences (such as cultural differences, insufficient or inappropriate instruction), they are not the result of those conditions or influences (National Joint Committee on Learning Disabilities, 1998; Swanson, 1991). Using a different definition, Torgesen (2002) described learning disabilities as problems acquiring academic knowledge and skills that are caused by disorders in basic psychological processes. These disorders are caused by a dysfunction of the central nervous system (CNS) that restricts cognitive functioning (Torgesen, 2002). Essentially, the LD brain receives and processes information differently from an intact brain. It is important to emphasise that a learning disability does not imply learning does not take place. Instead, it suggests that children with learning disabilities learn or demonstrate their knowledge in a manner different from that of their peers (Anglada, 2010).

Although learning disabilities initially concern performance in academic subjects, the ramifications of the disability extend into other spheres of the child's life (Bender & Wall, 1994; Siperstein, Bopp, & Bak, 1978). In addition to academic problems, empirical research suggests that children with LD are significantly more at risk of developing social and behavioural problems than their non-LD peers (Attah, 2010; Caletti & McLaughlin, 2003; Mishna & Muskat, 2004; Nowicki, 2003). For example, it is well documented that children with learning disabilities present with low social skills (Gresham, Sugai, & Horner, 2001; Swanson & Malone, 1992; Vaughn, Elbaum, & Boardman, 2001) and high rates of behaviour problems compared to their non-LD counterparts(Vaughn, Zaragoza, Hogan & Walker, 1993).

Although children with LDs may be common in Ghanaian schools (Yekple & Avoke, 2006), very little is known about their impact on academic achievement and behavior (Attah, 2010). In this chapter, we attempt to understand LD based on what has already been established. We start with an overview of how LD emerged as a field of study and subsequently how it developed in Ghana. Then, we explore the possible link between LD and academic achievement in Ghana. After that, we review how LD could be identified using culturally sensitive measures in Ghana schools. Later, we discuss the impact of LDs in relation to social skills and behavior problems. We conclude by offering recommendations for further research and good practice.

The history of learning disabilities

Learning disabilities (LD) is not a new concept. Its origins can be traced in the United States as far back as the early 1800s (Covington, 2004; Hallahan & Mercer, 2002). Early research studies had been keenly interested in how injuries to the brain affected adult functioning (Hinshelwood, 1917; Orton, 1937; Strauss & Kephart, 1955; Strauss & Lehtinen, 1947; Strauss & Werner, 1943). This interest stimulated an enormous amount of research that led to the evolution of the field labeled learning disabilities.

The earliest recognition of LD is assumed to have occurred in 1802. This was attributed to the work of Franz Joseph Gall, a German anatomist and physiologist. Gall explored the relationship between brain injury and mental impairment based on observations he had made of brain-injured soldiers (Carlson, 2005). He observed that some of these soldiers lacked speech but were still able to provide their thoughts in writing; this revealed a prototype of skill and deficits in oral and written language. Gall postulated that this outcome was a function of brain damage, the fact that a particular language capability was impaired due to injury whereas other abilities functioned normally. Continuing research advanced the study of brain areas associated with speech and language.

In the first quarter of the 20th century, there was a growing interest in the causes of reading disorders in individuals of normal intelligence. For example, James Hinshelwood (1917), an ophthalmologist, investigated a condition he later categorized as congenital word blindness (Hallahan & Kauffman, 1997; Lerner, 2000). Hinshelwood had observed that a congenital lesion in the left angular gyrus impaired the ability to store and recall visual memory of letters and words. This he found to be consistent among a group of people who had severe reading problems, but seemed otherwise intelligent without obvious visual impairments. He concluded that defective brain functions were responsible for the reading difficulties because he had seen the same type of problems in adults with brain tumours (Steenken, 2000).

Samuel Orton (1937), a specialist in neurology, extended the study of reading disabilities in his clinical studies. The studies were designed to test the hypothesis that reading deficits were a function of a delay or failure of the left cerebral hemisphere to establish dominance for language functions (Lyon, Fletcher, & Barnes, 2003). His findings were similar to that of Hinshelwood in that he observed in children with reading difficulties, the reversal of symbols, such as b and d, of words, such as saw and was (Kaufman, 2008). Orton drew the conclusion that the reading problems stemmed from disorders of memory. Both Hinshelwood and Orton presumed brain damage or dysfunction was tied directly to specific language disorders. Hence, they advocated assessment methods that strongly favoured remediation for children, specifically interventions that were aimed at improving reading and spelling deficits (Hallahan & Mercer, 2002; Hill, 1990; Kaufman, 2008; Lyon, Fletcher, & Barnes, 2003).

The work of Orton and Hinshelwood has been influential in shaping the LD field, and also in introducing descriptions of and interventions for reading disabilities (Lyon, et al., 2003). Contrary to the Orton and Hinshelwood approach, other researchers (Goldstein, Werner & Strauss) assumed that brain dysfunction found in persons with reading disabilities was as a result of an underlying perceptual processing disorder. For instance, Goldstein (1942) studied brain-injured soldiers returning from World War I, over several years. In his studies, he reported that patients displayed a consistent group of behaviours; many were hyperactive, easily distracted, and unable to read or write (Covington, 2004; Hallahan & Mercer, 2002; Kaufman, 2008).

Subsequently, psychologist Heinz Werner and psychiatrist Alfred Strauss studied mentally retarded adolescents and observed the same kind of perceptual, mood, and learning disorders in this low-IQ population that Goldstein had found with brain-injured soldiers (Kaufman, 2008). Based on these findings, Werner and Strauss deduced that there was a distinction between mental retardation caused by brain injury and mental retardation that was familial. Further, they found that special education aimed at treating the observed perceptual and behavioural problems was effective with mental retardation due to brain injury but not with inherited mental retardation. This implied that some of these adolescents labelled mentally retarded were not retarded but rather shared some of the same symptoms with regard to learning difficulties (Colbert, Elkins, Gunn, Muspratt & Wyatt-Smith, 2007; Kaufman, 2008).

Research was extended to the study of children with average or near average intelligence. These studies included children with known brain damage, such as cerebral palsy (Cruickshank, Bice, & Wallen, 1957) and intriguingly, samples of children who evidenced learning and behaviour problems but did not show clinical signs of brain damage (Strauss & Kephart, 1955). The research outcome moved the field forward in a dramatic way. It led to the establishment of a learning and behaviour disability caused by minimal brain dysfunction (MBD) (i.e. not detectable through standard clinical procedures, but brain injury nonetheless) that was distinct from mental retardation (as cited in Kaufman, 2008). This label, MBD, described children who were not mentally retarded, hearing impaired or emotionally disturbed but had minimal brain damage (Duchan, 2001; Friend, 2008; Smith, 2007). However, Werner and Strauss were greatly criticized for their deductions, because there was no scientific evidence to support that brain damage existed in such children. Additionally, their reasoning was based only on observable behaviour (Carlson, 2005). Nonetheless, the work of Werner and Strauss was further developed by Dolphin and William Cruikshank in the 1950s. William Cruikshank was one of the behavioural scientists who propelled the field away from a focus on etiology toward an emphasis on learner characteristics and educational interventions to address learning deficits (Hallahan & Mercer, 2002). During the formative years of LD research, from approximately 1939 to 1960, there was a paucity of research, very limited personnel, and no teacher education specifically oriented to LD as a discrete educational field. It was not until the early 1960s that a general awareness of this distinct group of children began to develop. Change came as a result of the pressure from parent groups who called for more educational attention to address the needs of the learning disabled. In addition, they stressed the need for a better definition (Bradford, Gottlieb & Zinkus, 1973). Parent groups had raised objections to the use of the labels "brain injury" and "minimally brain damaged" in addressing such children because of the condition of permanence it seemed to imply. Some professionals also claimed that it had little value in the classification, description and teaching of children (Hallahan & Mercer, 2002).

In 1963, as part of an effort to move away from a medical conceptualization, Kirk introduced the term "learning disability" whilst addressing a group of concerned parents in Chicago. The meeting was to discuss the special needs of their children (Dombrowski, Kamphaus & Reynolds, 2004; Hallahan & Kauffman, 1982; Hallahan & Mercer, 2002; Lerner, 1993; Lyon, Fletcher, & Barnes, 2003). The term learning disabilities as defined by Kirk referred to a disorder in which one or more of the psychological processes involved in understanding or using language, spoken, or written, manifest in an imperfect ability to listen, think, speak, read, write, spell, or do mathematical calculations. Children excluded from the definition were those who had learning problems which were primarily the result of visual, hearing, or motor handicaps, of mental retardation, of emotional disturbance, or of environmental, cultural, or economic disadvantage (Swanson & Willis, 1979).

The term learning disabled was accepted and endorsed by the parents (Mercer, 1982) who later established the parent organization Association of Children with Learning Disabilities (ACLD) and began to make demands no the US government for their children's needs to be met. Kirk's LD definition was from an educational perspective, focusing on the nature of the problem rather than on the hypothesized cause. Consequently, it served as the precursor for the US federal definitions and laws of the late 1960s and 1970s that proclaimed specific learning disabilities as a disorder that entitled special education services to anyone with a Specific Learning Disability diagnosis (Kaufman, 2008). In sum, the field of learning disabilities emerged with an aim to provide services to learning disabled students who were not being adequately served by the general educational system (Lyon, 1996; Lyon, Fletcher, & Barnes, 2003).

Learning disabilities in Ghana

In Ghana, a review of the literature reveals no clarity in how this concept of LD developed. Much of the literature available appears to have historical records on other special education categories (i.e.

sensory impairments, physical impairments, and mental retardation) but not on LD (Avoke, 2001). Before the arrival of special education in Ghana in 1954, exceptional children had been discriminated against. Children with disabilities were treated with hostility and rejection. Most of the arguments concerning the causes of disability were couched in religious and even superstitious terms (Avoke, 2001,). Many of these beliefs and attitudes were largely based on ignorance, misconception, misinformation and lack of appropriate education on the matter (Babalola, 2006).

Nonetheless, church organizations, missionary bodies, and non-governmental organizations (NGOs) were noted to have facilitated the establishment of special education services. The Special Education Division (SpEd) of the Ghana Education Service (GES) was set up in 1985 (Anthony, 2009). Over the years, they have been assisted by other related agencies (i.e. Ministry of Education, Science, and Sports (MOESS), the Assessment and Resource centers). However, special education services have narrowly focused on well-known special needs categories (i.e. visually impaired, hearing impaired, mental retardation etc.).

It is noted, although exact figures are unavailable, that child referrals due to persistent poor academic achievement are common in clinical settings (e.g. the Clinical Psychology Unit of the Psychiatry Hospital, Adabraka, the Psychiatry Department, University of Ghana Medical School, Korle Bu and others). Quite a number of these cases might not fall into any of the popular special needs categories mentioned above but instead meet LD diagnostic criteria.

Academic achievement and learning disabilities

There is evidence from a few Ghanaian studies that a proportion of children are not performing well in school. For instance, Wilmot (2001) found that 450 pupils from five randomly selected Ghanaian schools performed poorly in mathematics achievement measures. Low mathematics achievement was evident across sampled class levels (Class 3, 4 and 6). Similarly, in a related study, a large proportion of Ghanaian children were unable to read or write at an acceptable level. This was the observed trend across all grade levels (Kniel & Kniel,

2007). Likewise, results from the National Education Assessment (NEA - an indicator of Ghana's education quality at the basic level, 2007) revealed that less than 25% of Ghana's youth reach proficiency levels for English, and 10% attain proficiency in mathematics (Ministry of Education Sports and Science, 2008). Drawing from these studies, difficulties with school performance appear to be a problem in Ghana. While many factors could account for this, learning disabilities have been identified as one of the common reasons in Ghana (Yekple & Avoke, 2006).

Prevalence of learning disabilities

Globally, 5 percent or more of the school-age population experience difficulties with reading, mathematics and other skills that impede academic achievement (Fletcher et al., 2001; Lagae, 2008). Overall, in Ghana available information about the incidence of children with special needs is limited (MoESS, 2008) not to talk about specific categories such as LD. In the absence of studies, it is difficult to establish prevalence estimates. Nonetheless, for developing countries, Flisher, Malhotra, Nikopota and Patel (2008) have reported LD prevalence estimates that range between 2 percent and 10 percent of the child population. In Ghana, there is evidence indicating that LDs are predominant among school children although exact figures are lacking. For instance, Avoke and Yekple (2006) reported that learning disabilities were the most prevalent type of school-related problem among other impairments (i.e. hearing impairments, visual impairments) in Ghanaian schools. Similarly, in a study of four Ghanaian schools, Attah (2010) found that after ruling out other possible influences (e.g. hearing problems, visual problems) of academic difficulty, approximately 70% of the children assessed had one or more learning disability in reading, maths or spelling.

Identification of learning disabilities

From Western studies, it is noted that a variety of LD identification models exist, some of these are based on the assessment of IQ -achievement discrepancy, low achievement, impairment and neuropsychological deficits among others. A review of the literature in

Africa showed that most researchers (Babalola, 2006; Ikujuni, 2006; Lere, 2006; Yekple & Avoke, 2006) do not offer criteria on how LDs are assessed or identified. In the absence of standard guidelines to assess learning disabilities in Ghana, some professionals (e.g. psychologists, therapists, and teachers) have developed their own procedures. But, the scope of their work is a function of the resources available (King de Larrarte, 1993).Though not documented, the assessment of LD at the Clinical Psychology Unit of the Accra Psychiatry Hospital is based on low academic achievement (as measured by WRAT), average or above average non-verbal intelligence (as measured by Ravens Progressive Matrices) and adaptive behaviour skills. Consistent with the NJCLD definition of LD, the possibility of mental retardation, emotional imbalance, visual impairment, hearing impairments as causes for low achievement has to be ruled out. However, these decisive factors are vaguely defined and may vary in how they are established from one clinician to another.

In an attempt to develop a quick screening procedure for identifying LD in Ghana, Attah (2010) demonstrated that *a neurological screening test, non-verbal intelligence and adaptive behavior measures* (with Ghanaian norms) could be used to differentiate children with LD from other children (e.g. mental retardation, cerebral palsy etc.) with learning difficulties. These measures proved to be culturally sensitive for identifying school children with LD.

The impact of learning disabilities

Ghanaians value academic achievement as evidenced by the efforts of government to enhance student academic performance (Ampiah, Davis & Mankoe, 2006; Etsey, 2005; Gerhart, 2007; Katsiyannis, Zhang, Ryan & Jones, 2007). Parents begin to reinforce their children's academic capabilities at a very young age, because of the strong competition that seems to persist in the educational sector. Hence, children are under a lot of pressure at school to perform (Tzeng, 2007). With such high value placed on academic skills in society, the child who fails to achieve as expected may develop feelings of personal inadequacy and become frustrated. For parents, a child's poor academic performance can be very frustrating as some invest a great deal of money in their child's education.

In Ghana for instance, basic education is free. Although statistics are not available, the majority of parents spend extra money for extra classes (arranged privately at home or by the schools throughout the week) to ensure that their wards are successful in school. Despite this, many children still struggle with school work as their educational needs may not have been addressed appropriately. Children with LD are likely to fall into this category because teachers are sometimes unaware they have a disability. Even if they are aware, many teachers lack the requisite skills to deal with problems associated with LD. Unfortunately, such children may progress from class to class unnoticed or be retained in the same class without promotion. For instance, over half of the students identified with LD in Attah's study (2010) had repeated one class or more due to poor performance. The truth is, few attempts are made to find causative factors for their academic failure (Sharma, 2004). Commonly, parents, teachers and peers are likely to assume that the child with LD is lazy, slow or unintelligent (Broatch, 2004). Many, students who are not able to cope may change schools, drop out of school or become truants (Agbenyega, 2003). Drawing from this, a unique section of the Ghanaian school populace might have an LD that has not been identified.

Specifically, in Western literature, it has been hypothesized that as a consequence of school failure, parents, teachers, and peers express disapproval of the child in question. Such response could lead to further academic failure and subsequent social and emotional problems (Bruck, 1986). It is thus not surprising that in Attah's (2010) study, students with LD presented with poor social skills and a range of particular behavioral problems. In this study, it was found that children with LD were more likely to overestimate their own abilities, react poorly to criticism, poorly to frustration, demand excessive attention or praise, seem to feel persecuted, have hypochondriacal tendencies and show other signs of emotional instabilities compared with children without LD. These behavioural patterns highlight typical problems a Ghanaian LD child is likely to experience.

The way forward

From the little that has been established, LD is a valid area of study that requires further research in Ghana. Although it is important to learn from Western studies to enhance our understanding of LD, there is an urgent need to advance LD research in our cultural setting as the needs and focus of remediation may differ. Research aimed at identifying affected populations (e.g. children, adolescent and adult), and establishing prevalence patterns should be encouraged. As we begin to gain a better understanding of LD in Ghana, we should aim to develop culturally sensitive treatment programmes for children with LD.

It would be important for teacher's to play a proactive role in referring children with academic, social and behavioural problems for psychological assessment. Since LDs are not visually obvious, social skill deficits or behavioural problems could hint at underlying LD. Although this may not be true for all cases, a qualified psychologist should be able to confirm the presence of an LD, and identify problem areas that would require remediation. Also, educators should be trained to realize that LD students learn differently, thus the mode of instruction should be adapted to meet their specific learning needs.

Research in this area is yet to receive its due recognition in Ghana. The absence of solid research implies an unawareness of LD as a subject of special importance. Professionals, educators and researchers alike are desperately needed to further advance the knowledge obtained in the current study. In the words of Carlson (2005, p.17), "Without caring and inquisitive people willing to seek out new horizons, there can be no new intervention theories. We have come a long way, but we are not there yet".

References

Abosi O. (2007). Educating Children with Learning Disabilities in Africa. *Learning Disabilities Research & Practice,* 22 (3), 196–201.

Agbenyega, J. (2003, December). The power of labeling discourse in the construction of disability in Ghana. In *A* paper presented at the Australian Association for Research in Education Conference, Newcastle, Association of Active Educational Researchers (AARE).

Ampiah J. G., Davis, E. K. & Mankoe, J. O. (2006). An Investigation of Provision of Quality Basic Education in Ghana A Case Study of Selected Schools in the Central Region.

Anglada, T. (2010). When Learning is the Problem. *Pediatrics for Parents*, 26, 25-27.

Anthony, J. H.(2009). Access to Education for Students with Autism in Ghana: Implications for EFA. A Commissioned Background Report Prepared for the Global Monitoring Report, 2010.

Avoke, M. (2001). Some Historical Perspectives in the development of Special Education in Ghana. *European Journal of Special Needs Education,* 16 (1), 29-40.

Attah, D. A.(2010). Learning Disabilities and Academic Achievement among School Children in Accra. University of Ghana, Legon Thesis (Unpublished).

Babalola, G. O. (2006). An Assessment of Special Education Practices in Nigeria: A Shift from Initiation of Schools to Inclusive Education. *African Journal of Special Educational Needs*, IV, 306-315.

Bender,W. N., & Wall,M. (1994). Social-emotional development of students with learning disabilities. *Learning Disabilities Quarterly, 17,* 323–341.

Bradford L. J., Gottlieb M. I. & Zinkus (1979). Current issues in Developmental Pediatrics: The Learning – Disabled Child. New York:Stratton,

Broatch, L. (2004). Learning Disabilities and Psychological Problems-An Overview. *A Parent's Guide to Psychological Problems.* 1- 4.

Bruck, M. (1986). Social and emotional adjustments of learning disabled children: A review of the issues. In S.J. Ceci (Ed.), *Handbook of Cognitive, Social and Neuropsychological Aspects of Learning Disabilities* 1, 361-380.

Caletti, C. M. & McLaughlin T. F. (2003) The Social-Behavioral Difficulties Associated with Nonverbal Learning Disabilities: Some Suggestions for Educators; *International Journal of Special Education. 18 (1) 55-66.*

Carlson S. (2005). A Two Hundred Year History of Learning Disabilities. A Research Document, Regis University.

Colbert, Elkins, Gunn, Muspratt & Wyatt-Smith, (2007). Literature Review. Changing the nature of support provision. *Student with learning difficulties: Interventions in literacy and numeracy project (InLaN).* 2, 1-225.

Collins, D. W., & Rourke, B. P. (2003). Learning-disabled brains: A review of the literature. *Journal of Clinical and Experimental Neuropsychology, 25,* 1011-1034.

Covington, L. E. (2004). Moving Beyond the Limits of Learning: Implications of Learning Disabilities for Adult Education. *Journal of Adult Basic Education* 14, 90-103.

Cowardin, N. (1998). Disorganized Crime: Learning Disability and the criminal justice system, *Criminal Justice*, 13, 11-16.

Cruickshank, W. M., Bice, H. V., & Wallen, N. E. (1957). *Perception and cerebral palsy.* Syracuse: Syracuse University Press.

Dombrowski, S. C., Kamphaus, R. W., & Reynolds, C. R. (2004). After the demise of the discrepancy: Proposed learning disability diagnostic criteria. *Professional Psychology:Research and Practice, 35,* 364–372.

Duchan, J. (2001). History of speech-pathology in America: Kurt Goldstein. Available at: e eb:http://www.ascu.buffalo.edu/~duchan/historysub-pages. Dtae accessed 9 November, 2005.

Etsey, K. (2005). Causes of low academic performance of primary school pupils in the Shama Sub-Metro of Shama Ahanta East Metropolitan Assembly (SAEMA) in Ghana. Present at the Regional Conference on Education in West Africa Dakar, Senegal. *Exceptional Children, 42*, 136-144.

Flisher, A. J., Malhotra S., Nikapota A. & Patel V. (2008). Promoting child and adolescent mental health in low and middle income countries. *Journal of Child Psychology and Psychiatry* 49:3 313–334.

Friend, M. (2008). Special Education: Contemporary Perspectives for School Professionals, Second Edition. Allyn & Bacon/Longman.

Gerhart, G. M. (2007). *The New Book of Knowledge*. Danbury: Scholastic Library Publishing.

Goldstein, K. (1942). *After- effects of brain injuries in war.* New York: Grune & Stratton.

Gresham, F. M., Sugai & Horner, R. H. (2001).Interpreting outcomes of social skillstraining for students with high-incidents disabilities.‘ *The Council for Exceptional Children*, 67, 331– 44.

Hallahan D. P. & Kauffman, J. M. (1982). Exceptional Children (2nd edition). Introduction to Special Education. Prentice-Hall, Inc, Englewood.

Hallahan, D.P. & Kauffman, J.M. (1997). Exceptional children: Introduction to special education (7th ed.). Boston: Allyn and Bacon.

Hallahan, D. P. & Mercer, C. D. (2002). Learning disabilities: Historical perspectives.

In: Bradley, R., Danielson, L., & Hallahan, D.P. (Eds.). Identification of Learning Disabilities: Research to Practice. Mahwah, New Jersey: Lawrence Erlbaum Associates.

Hill, J. (1990). The Learning Disabled and the Public School Programs. A thesis submitted to Broward Community College.

Hinshelwood, J. (1917). *Congenital word blindness.* London: H. K. Lewis. Hinshelwood, J. (1895). Word- blindness and visual memory. *Lancet, 2,* 1564– 1570.

Interagency Committee on Learning Disabilities. (1987). Learning disabilities: A report to the U. S. Congress. Washington DC: U. S. Department of Health and Human Services.

Katsiyannis, A. Zhang, D. Ryan, J. B. & Jones, J. (2007). High-Stakes Testing and Students with Disabilities: Challenges and Promises *Journal of Disability Policy Studies*, 18, 160-167.

Kaufman, A. S. (2008). Neuropsychology and Specific Learning Disabilities: Lessons from the Past as a Guide to Present Controversies and Future Clinical Practice. Neuropsychological Perspectives on Learning Disabilities in the Era of RTI: Recommendations for Diagnosis and Intervention. Fletcher-Janzen, E., & Reynolds, C.R. (Eds), 1-13.

King De Larrarte, C. I. (1993). Learning Disabilities in Colombia, South America. *Journal of Learning Disabilities,* 26, 499-500.

Kniel, A. & Kniel,C. (2007). Ghana Adaptive Behavior Scale. An Assessment tool to measure competence in daily life of Ghanaian children. German Technical Cooperation.

Lagae, L. (2008). Learning disabilities: definitions, epidemiology, diagnosis, and intervention strategies. *Pediatric Clinics of North America*, 55(6), 1259-1268.

Lerner J. W. (1993). Learning Disabilities: Theories, Diagnosis, and Teaching Strategies. Houghton Mifflin Company.

Lerner, J. W. (2000). Learning Disabilities: Theories, Diagnosis and Teaching Strategies. 8th ed. Boston, MA: Houghton Mifflin Company.

Lyon, G. R., Fletcher, J. M., & Barnes, M. C. (2003). Learning disabilities. In E. J. Mash & R. A. Barkley (Eds.), *Child psychopathology,* (2nd ed.) 520-586.

Mash, E. J. & Wolfe, D. A. (2007). *Abnormal Child Psychology*. 3ed. Wadsworth a division of Thomson Learning, Inc.

Ministry of Education Sports & Science (MoESS) (2008), Preliminary Education Sector Performance Report, Ministry of Education, Science & Sports, Accra, Ghana, 51.

Mishna F. & Muskat, B. (2004). School- Based Group Treatment for Students with Learning Disabilities: A Collaborative Approach. *Journal of Children and Schools*. 26, 135 – 150.

National Joint Committee on Learning Disabilities (1998). Operationalizing the NJCLD definition of learning disabilities for ongoing assessment in the schools. *Learning Disabilities Quarterly, 21*, 186–193.

Nowicki, E. (2003). A meta-analysis of the social competence of children with learning disabilities compared to classmates of low and average to high achievement. *Learning Disability Quarterly, 26*(3), 171-188.

Orton, S. T. (1937). *Reading, writing, and speech problems in children.* New York: W. W. Norton & Company, Inc.

Sharma, G. (2004). A Comparative Study of the Personality Characteristics of Primary- School Students with Learning Disabilities and their Non Learning Disabled Peers. Learning Disability Quartely, 27, 127-139.

Siperstein, G. N., Bopp, M., & Bak, J. (1978). Social status of learning disabled children. *Journal of Learning Disabilities*, 11, 49-53.

Smith D. D. (2007) Introduction to Special Education: Making a Difference. Learning Disabilities. Allyn & Bacon/Longman.

Steenken E. M. (2000). Having a Learning Disability: It's Effect on the Academic Decisions of College Students. A dissertation submitted to the faculty of the Virginia Polytechnic Institute State University.

Strauss, A. A., & Kephart, N. C. (1955). *Psychopathology and education of the brain- injured child* New York: Grune & Stratton.

Strauss, A. A., & Lehtinen, L. E. (1947). *Psychopathology and education of the brain- injured child. Volume 2: Progress in theory and clinic.* New York: Grune & Stratton.

Strauss, A. A., & Werner, H. (1943). Comparative psychopathology of the brain- injured child and the traumatic brain- injured adult. *American Journal of Psychiatry, 99*, 835– 838.

Swanson, H. L. (1991). Operational definitions and learning disabilities: An overview. *Learning Disability Quarterly, 14*, 242–254. Published by: Council for Learning Disabilities Stable URL: http://www.jstor.org/stable/1510661.

Swanson, H. L & Malone, S. (1992). Social skills and learning disabilities: A meta- analysis of the literature. *School Psychology Review.* 21, 427-443.

Swanson, B. M. & Willis, D. J. (1979). Children with Specific Learning Disabilities. Understanding Exceptional Children and Youth: An

Introduction to Special Education. Chicago:Rand McNally College Publishing Company.

Tanner, D. E. (2001). The Learning Disabled: A Distinct Population of Students. *Journal of Education.* 121(4), 795-798.

Torgesen, J. K. (2002). Empirical and theoretical support for direct diagnosis of learning disabilities by assessment of intrinsic processing weaknesses. In R. Bradley, L. Danielson, & D. Hallahan (Eds.), *Identification of learning disabilities: Research to practice* (pp. 565-650). Mahwah, NJ: Lawrence Erlbaum. Associates, Inc.

Tzeng, S-J. (2007). Learning Disabilities in Taiwan: A Case of Cultural Constraints on the Education of Students with Disabilities. *Learning Disabilities Research & Practice,22,* 170–175.

Vaughn, S., Elbaum, B. & Boardman A. G. (2001). The Social Functioning of Students With Learning Disabilities: Implications for Inclusion. *Exceptionality,* 9(1&2), 47–65.

Vaughn, S., Zaragoza, N., Hogan A. & Walker J. (1993). A Four-Year Longitudinal Investigation of Social Skills and Behavior Problems of Students with Learning Disabilities. *Journal of Learning Disabilities.* 26(6), 404-412.

Wilmot, E. M. (2001). Gender Differences in Mathematics Achievement in Primary Schools in Ghana. *Mathematics Connection*, 2, 25-29.

Yekple, Y. E. (2008). The role of the Teacher in meeting the divergent needs of children in the classroom. *African Journal of Special Education*, V, 184-192.

Yekple, Y. E. & Avoke, M. (2006). Improving Inclusive Education at Basic School Level in Ghana. *African Journal of Special needs.* IV (2), 239 -249.

Chapter 19
Dilemmas of Healthcare Professionals in Ghana

Angela Ofori-Atta and Helen Jack

Introduction

Health care providers often face situations of ethical tension when caring for patients (Kass, 2001). The ways in which they manage ethical dilemmas affect the care they provide, their relationship with patients, and their own morale. Ethical or moral dilemmas are complex situations that often involve an apparent conflict between moral imperatives and that are underpinned by the normative ethical principles of beneficence, non-maleficence, respect for the autonomy of others, and utility (net balance of benefits over harm).

The recognition that healthcare professionals will act differently in situations based on their ethno-religious, personal, and socio-cultural backgrounds has prompted an unprecedented level of attention being paid to ethical dimensions in clinical practice in high-income countries (Haas & Fennimore, 1983). Multiple studies document and classify ethical dilemmas, many of which depend on the specific legal or cultural context in which the professionals are working (Battaglia, Epstein, and Roberts, 1999; Raines, 2000). For instance, Wilkinson (1988) describes dilemmas arising from issues related to prolonging life, the performance of unnecessary tests, and the desire to speak truth (Wilkinson,1988). Cash (2005) included a lack of access to drugs and good health care facilities leading to a denial of the basic rights of patients (Cash, 2005).

Facing ethical tension can cause increased stress and burnout among health care professionals (Raines, 2000; Kalvemark, 2003; Ulrich et al., 2007; Wlodarczyk & Lazarewicz, 2011), which can contribute to poor health (Dovlo, 2005) and, in a low-resource setting, could contribute to brain drain. Education in medical ethics can equip health care professionals with skills to analyze ethical situations and a moral foundation on which to base decision-making (Eckles et al., 2005) and may reduce stress related to ethical dilemmas (Folmar et al., 1997). To most effectively help health care professionals handle situations of ethical tension, ethics education must be tailored to the types of scenarios and decisions that health care professionals are confronting (Bissonette et al., 1995). Although understanding the ethical dilemmas that health care professionals face is fundamental to designing robust training programmes in medical ethics, we are aware of no studies that have examined the ethical dilemmas of health care professionals in a low-medium- income country (LMIC).

A better understanding of the ethical dilemmas of health care professionals in Ghana could inform the design of training in medical ethics that could help Ghana's health care professionals more effectively navigate situations of ethical tension. Accordingly, we sought to explore the experiences of Ghanaian health care professionals with ethical dilemmas to gain a deeper understanding of the ethical choices medical professionals face.

Methods

Study design and sample

For a class assignment in psychiatry in February 2012, final year medical students at the University of Ghana Medical School were each asked to interview one health care professional about his or her most difficult ethical dilemma. Complete descriptive information is displayed in Figure 6.

The University of Ghana Medical School's Ethics Committee approved all research procedures

Data collection

In order to promote candour among respondents, the medical students carried out semi-structured, open-ended interviews, asking respondents to describe their most difficult ethical dilemma and how they resolved it (McCracken, 1996). The sample size was determined based on the number of medical students in the course; each student interviewed one health care professional. The medical students collected basic demographic information about the respondents then took hand-written notes during the interview and typed up a summary of the dilemma and its resolution following the interview.

Data analysis

During an initial review of the dilemmas, the researchers inductively developed a list of common scenarios—situations of ethical tension that multiple healthcare professionals face. One researcher (HJ) read through all of the dilemmas and created a list of common scenarios. If the researcher encountered a dilemma that did not fit into the list of of common scenarios, a new scenerio type was added to ensure that all possible scenarios were captured (Glaser & Strauss, 1967). After all dilemmas were coded, any scenarios that had only one dilemma were grouped in an "Other" category. Additionally, because the common scenario analysis showed that the patient's families were involved in many dilemmas, the researcher counted the number of dilemmas in which the patient's family played a major role, defined as when the dilemma forced the health care professional to consider not only the patient's interests, but also the interests of the family.

Next, we reviewed existing classification systems for ethical decisions in health care (Battaglia, Epstein, & Roberts, 1999; Raines, 2000; Callahan & Jennings, 2002; Baum et al., 2009) and, based on an existing classification system (Baum et al., 2009), designed a broad classification system that would capture the themes in our data and that was appropriate for use in a LMIC setting. The researchers separately reviewed each dilemma report and placed it into one of the four classification categories. They compared their classifications, recorded the number of discrepant assignments, and reconciled their classifications through discussion.

Results

The interviewees (n=153) were primarily physicians (n=122) or nurses (n=17) and ranged in age from 24 to 76 years. They had been working in a variety of areas of medicine when the ethical dilemma occurred, including obstetrics and gynaecology, paediatrics, general medicine, surgery, and infectious disease. Table 19.1 presents complete descriptive information of the sample.

Table 19.1: Descriptive characteristics of health care providers

Descriptive factor	Subjects
Gender	Male: 97 Female: 30 Unlisted: 24
Area of medicine (top 5)	Obstetrics and Gynecology: 56 Paediatrics: 29 General: 23 Surgery: 16 Infectious Disease: 10
Age range	24-76
Position	Physician: 122 Nurse: 17 Resident: 8 Pharmacist: 1 Dentist: 1 Medical Assistant: 1 Medical Student: 1

Common scenarios for dilemmas

The seven most common scenarios involved patient refusal of blood transfusions due to religious beliefs, patient confidentiality versus family members' requests for information, patients' rights to refuse care, conflict of values of professionals with respect to abortion, resource limitations and lying for a patient. If the two categories of limitation of resources (institutional vs patient resources) were merged, then resource limitations would constitute the second largest category (17%) equal to sharing of information with families (i.e. keeping patient confidentiality).

Examining these common scenarios further showed that 32 percent of the dilemmas involved the patient's family (48 cases), including all dilemmas related to sharing information and HIV status and some dilemmas related to abortion, refusal of care, fertility, and negligence. Table 19.2 displays complete descriptions of the common scenarios and the number of dilemmas classified in each scenario.

Table 19.2: Common scenarios for the dilemmas of health care providers

Scenario	Number of dilemmas
Adult Jehovah's Witness: What to do when a patient refuses a blood transfusion because he or she is a Jehovah's Witness	18
Sharing information: Whether to share information about a patient's condition with the patient's family or guardians	17
HIV status: Whether to disclose a patient's HIV status to the patient's family	15
Patient refuses care: What to do when patient refuses to follow medical advice	15
Abortion: Whether to perform an abortion if the procedure goes against the provider's religious or moral principles	12
Resource shortage: What to do when a lack of resources on the part of a patient or a patient's inability to pay make providing care difficult	11
Lying: Whether to lie at the request of a patient	10
Negligence: Whether to tell hospital staff and/or a patient's family about the negligence of another medical provider	9
Fertility: Whether to preserve a woman's fertility when it puts the woman's life at greater risk	9
Jehovah's Witness (child): What to do when the family of a minor refuses to consent for the minor to have a blood transfusion because they are Jehovah's Witnesses	9
Resource shortage: Unavailable or limited institutional material or human resource	6
Assisted suicide: Whether or not to help a patient die when the patient or the patient's family has requested assistance	3
Patient violence: How to behave when patients act aggressively	2
Poor prognosis: Whether to perform a procedure on a patient who has a poor prognosis	2
Other	13

Classification of dilemmas

The researchers classified each dilemma into one of four broad categories:

Determining appropriate use of authority: Health care professionals faced decisions about when to limit the freedom, autonomy, or confidentiality of a patient or the patient's family. They had to decide, for example, whether to treat a child contrary to the wishes of the parents or whether to disclose a patient's positive HIV status to that person's sexual partner.

Making decisions about resource allocation: Health care professionals had to decide how to allocate scarce human or physical resources, including their own time, between individuals, groups, populations, or programmes. For example, one physician had only one unit of a blood type that two patients, one poor and one wealthy, needed, and he had to decide to whom to give the blood.

Ensuring standards of quality of care: Health care professionals, faced with limited resources or programme constraints that would force them to provide lower quality care, had to choose how to proceed and what sacrifices to make. For example, nurses and physicians had to decide whether to carry out a procedure they had little experience doing and feared they would do poorly when there were no specialist professionals available to perform the procedure.

Questioning the role or scope of the health care professional: The views of health care professionals differed from those of their patients or the patients' families with regard to the role of health care professional and what services healthcare professionals should be providing to the individual or the community. For example, physicians struggled with the decision about whether to perform an abortion when it was against their moral or religious beliefs, but the woman requested it.

The two most common categories of dilemmas for healthcare workers were *Determining the appropriate use of authority* and *Questioning the role or scope of the health care professional*. The distribution of dilemmas between classifications is displayed in Table 19.3 and Figure 19.1.

Table 19.3: Classification of dilemmas

Classification	Number of dilemmas
Determining appropriate use of authority	68
Making decisions about resource allocation	12
Ensuring standards of quality of care	11
Questioning the role or scope of the health care professional	60

Fig 19.1 **Distribution of dilemma classifications**

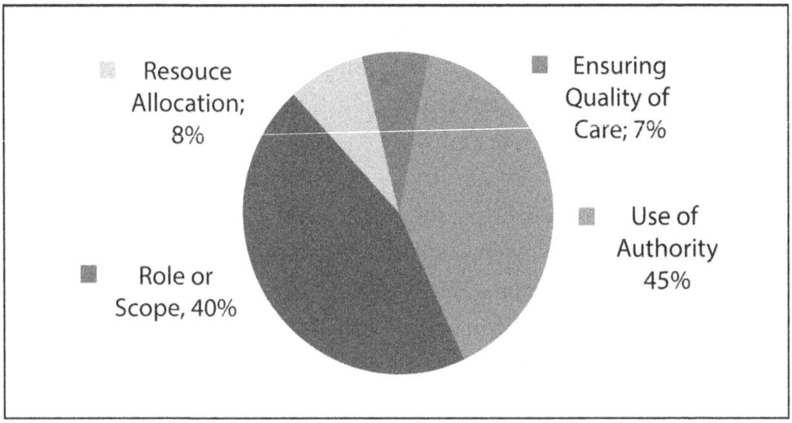

Discussion

The results show that one-third of dilemmas involve the families of patients, an aspect of ethical dilemmas that has not been highlighted by previous studies. Existing research on ethical dilemmas of health care professionals has not emphasized the role of the family (Battaglia, Epstein, and Roberts, 1999; Raines, 2000). The finding about the role of family may be specific to a Ghanaian or LMIC context where traditional family structure and communal culture are highly valued and where limited resources necessitate that family play a greater role in patient care. Ghanaian households may be large and span many generations, leading to close family ties, interdependencies, and a defined family hierarchy. Additionally, the families of patients often play a large role in their care, bringing them food, leaving the hospital to get necessary medications, and monitoring the patient when hospital staff are not available. A single ethical case study from India highlights the role of the family in ethical dilemmas, showing that this pattern may also exist in other LMICs (Gopichandrann & Gaitonde, 2011).

The code of the Ghana Medical Association dictates that the physician must consider the family's interests, but that the wishes of the patient take precedence (Manual of the Ghana Medical Association). Additionally, Ghana's Patient's Bill of Rights and other legal documents provide specific guidelines on how to negotiate many dilemmas where the patient's autonomy is in question (Ghana Patient's Bill of Rights). If physicians were aware of these regulations and empowered to take an active role in overriding family hierarchy to protect the patient's best interests, they may feel more prepared to handle these situations. Ethics education could play a role in informing health care professionals about existing guidelines and providing a space for them to discuss how to enforce those principles in the midst of interpersonal and cultural pressures.

Additionally, the results indicate that 85 percent of dilemmas are related to determining the appropriate use of authority or the role and scope of the health care professional. Consistent with the classification results, previous studies have emphasized the predominance of dilemmas that involve questions about authority or role of the medical professional (Baum et al., 2009). These classification results demonstrate that Ghanaian health professionals take patient values into consideration, a notable finding in Ghana's traditionally hierarchical and paternalistic society.

Although Ghana was until recently, a low-income country and medical professionals work within a resource-limited health system, few dilemmas were related to the lack or allocation of resources. One possible explanation is that patients who have severely limited resources do not present for care or they leave care when faced with high costs, giving healthcare professionals few opportunities to interact with them. Further research is needed to explore whether this is because health care professionals face these dilemmas so frequently that they no longer consider them challenging, they have training or procedures that prepare them to handle these situations, or they rarely encounter such dilemmas. Ethics training may not need to focus on questions of resources, but could alert professionals that some patients become invisible because they do not return for treatment due to lack of resources, and highlight ways health care professionals could follow-up with and assist these patients.

The findings of this study must be interpreted in the light of several limitations. First, there was some variation in the ways that dilemmas were gathered and reported because each was collected and summarized by a different student. In order to minimize reporting differences, the students were given the same instructions on questions to ask, data to report, and reporting format. Secondly, because this is a preliminary study on a topic about which little is known, the selection of respondents was not based on a representative sample of all medical professionals in Ghana. A larger, systematic study is needed to further explore the prevalence and distribution of the types of ethical dilemmas that health care professionals face. Furthermore, in order to understand the full scope of ethical decision making, it is necessary to explore a broader range of dilemmas, not only those that health care professionals consider most challenging, and to investigate how medical professionals are resolving situations of ethical tension. Fourthly, health care professionals may not have been open with the medical students, and more experienced and anonymous interviewers should be used in future studies.

This study reveals that health care professionals in Ghana often face ethical dilemmas related to their role, responsibility, and that many of those dilemmas involve weighing the wishes or best interest of the family against those of the patient. These findings can inform ethics education and further research on the dilemmas of health care professionals in low-income countries.

References

Baum, N. M., Gollust, S. E., Goold, S. D., & Jacobson, P. D. (2009). Ethical issues in public health practice in Michigan. *American Journal of Public Health,99* (2), 369.

Bissonette, R., O'Shea, R., Horwitz, M., & Rout, C. (1995). A data-generated basis for medical ethics education: Categorizing issues experienced by students during clinical training. *Acad Med, 70*(11), 1035-1037.

Callahan, D., & Jennings, B. (2002). Ethics and public health: Forging a strong relationship. *Journal Information, 92*(2).

Dovlo, D. (2007). Migration of nurses from Sub-Saharan Africa: A review of issues and challenges. *Health Services Research, 42*(3p2), 1373-1388.

Eckles, R. E., Meslin, E. M., Gaffney, M., & Helft, P. R. (2005). Medical ethics education: Where are we? where should we be going? A review. *Academic Medicine, 80*(12), 1143.

Eckles, R. E., Meslin, E. M., Gaffney, M., & Helft, P. R. (2005). Medical ethics education: Where are we? where should we be going? A review. *Academic Medicine, 80*(12), 1143.

Folmar, J., Coughlin, S. S., Bessinger, R., & Sacknoff, D. (1997). Ethics in public health practice: A survey of public health nurses in southern Louisiana. *Public Health Nursing, 14*(3), 156-160.

Glaser, B. G., & Strauss, A. L. (1967). *The discovery of grounded theory: Strategies for qualitative research.*

Gopichandran, V., & Gaitonde, R. (2011). When the patient's family refuses care: A practical ethical dilemma. *Indian Journal Medical Ethics*, 248-249.

Healy, T. C. (2003). Ethical decision making: Pressure and uncertainty as complicating factors. *Health & Social Work, 28*(4), 293-301.

Kälvemark, S., Höglund, A. T., Hansson, M. G., Westerholm, P., & Arnetz, B. (2004). Living with conflicts-ethical dilemmas and moral distress in the health care system. *Social Science & Medicine, 58*(6), 1075-1084.

Kass, N. E. (2001). An ethics framework for public health. *Journal Information, 91*(11)

Managing exits. (2006). *World Health Report 2006*, World Health Organization.

Raines, M. L. (2000). Ethical decision making in nurses: Relationships among moral reasoning, coping style, and ethics stress. *JONA'S Healthcare Law, Ethics and Regulation,* 2(1), 29&hyhen; 41.

Roberts, L. W., Battaglia, J., & Epstein, R. S. (1999). Frontier ethics: Mental health care needs and ethical dilemmas in rural communities. *Psychiatric Services, 50*(4), 497-503.

Ulrich, C., O'Donnell, P., Taylor, C., Farrar, A., Danis, M., & Grady, C. (2007). Ethical climate, ethics stress, and the job satisfaction of nurses and social workers in the united states. *Social Science & Medicine, 65*(8), 1708-1719.

Wlodarczyk, D., & Lazarewicz, M. (2011). Frequency and burden with ethical conflicts and burnout in nurses. *Nursing Ethics, 18*(6), 847-861.

Chapter 20

Experience of Strengthening the Mental Health Information System in Ghana's Three Psychiatric Hospitals

A.Ofori-Atta, T. Mirzoev, A. Mensah-Kufuor, A. Osei, A. Dzadey, K. Armah-Aloo, K.D.Atweam

Introduction

The World Health Organization defines a Mental Health Information System (MHIS) as 'a system for collecting, processing, analysing, disseminating and using information about a mental health service and the mental health needs of the population it serves (WHO, (2005). Developing MHIS may be considered a costly intervention, and yet the ultimate aim in establishing MHIS in low-income countries is for a more equitable distribution of resources in the context of scarcity (Husein, Adeyi, Bryant et al., 1993) . This is particularly pertinent for mental health care in Ghana, where there is inequitable distribution of mental health services (Doku, Ofori-Atta, Akpalu, et al., 2008).

A situation analysis of mental health policy implementation in Ghana was conducted as the first phase of the Mental Health and Poverty Project (MHAPP). The MHAPP was a 5-year (research consortium project funded by the Department for International Development of the United Kingdom (DfID) and it ended in December 2010. The situation analysis revealed numerous challenges faced by the existing Mental Health Information System (MHIS) in Ghana (Doku et al., 2008). There was limited information on mental health collected routinely at the three psychiatric hospitals, and the district and regional hospitals. The information also focused on four disease categories only (psychotic disorders, epilepsy, substance use disorders and neurosis). The definitions of the categories were not standardized across the different data-gathering institutions, results were poorly analysed, rarely disseminated and the output was not useful to policy makers or for mental health advocacy. In response to the above challenges, an intervention to strengthen the MHIS in Ghana was implemented with support from the MHAPP and in collaboration with the Ghana Health Service.

MHIS is owned by the Ministry of Health and the Ghana Health Service (GHS). This intervention was therefore a collaboration between the Ghana Health Service and the Mental Health and Poverty Project (MHAPP). A basic understanding to work conjointly towards the strengthening of the MHIS was agreed upon, with the MHAPP acting as collaborator and catalyst, and the Ministry of Health and its institutions as the implementers. The GHS provided the human resources, with the MHAPP contributing specialist and financial resources. The objective of this paper is to report on the design and implementation of the MHIS, and to deliberate on the factors which influenced these processes and the key intervention effects.

General principles on health management information systems which were considered in the design of the MHIS

Our design for the development of the MHIS was informed by general principles deduced from literature. The literature showed that challenges when developing health information systems generally in developing countries include insufficient training for staff responsible for implementation, lack of understanding of the changes introduced, inadequate supervision for staff involved, and lack of the skills and abilities necessary to undertake additional responsibilities required by the HMIS (Gladwin, Dixon, and Wilson, 2003) . Furthermore, systems must be 'user friendly' (WHO 2005) in order to have the best chance of consistent and accurate collection of data by health care workers (Husein et al., 1993). There is the need to focus on a broad spectrum of mental disorders, not only those for which treatment is available in order to illustrate unmet need so as to lobby for greater resources. One must also decide whether data collected should be population or facility-based depending on how comprehensive the data need to be (Kustner, Varo, and Gonzales, 2002). An MHIS that collects data only from mental health services is likely to exclude many cases. Finally, process issues such as consultation with stake-holders, and the need for monitoring and evaluation, are worth planning for (Odhiambo-Otieno, 2005a; Odhiambo-Otieno, 2005b).

Intervention design and implementation

Intervention design. The intervention was aimed to strengthen and expand MHIS at the psychiatric hospitals, focusing on the functions of collection, processing, analysis, and use of information. The MHIS was designed to include a combination of paper-based and computerized elements. Patients were given a registration form on each visit, which was filled in as they contacted professionals in each department of the hospital. On exit, the form was retained and sent to the records department, where it was entered into the database.

Sites: The intervention was implemented in the three state psychiatric hospitals providing both outpatient and inpatient care, and situated in the south of the country: Accra, Pantang and Ankaful psychiatric hospitals.

Intervention implementation: The implementation involved four broad aspects. Firstly, there was liaison between the Policy, Planning Monitoring and Evaluation Division (PPMED) of the GHS and a mandate was received by the MHAPP team to develop the existing MHIS at the three psychiatric hospitals, following an agreement on the changes considered feasible by the management and records departments of the three psychiatric hospitals. It was agreed that this would be the first part of a larger intervention to develop MHIS at the district and regional levels in order to ensure compatibility. Secondly, there was consultation which led to agreement on a standard set of diagnostic categories to be collected, and a uniform process for data collection in the three hospitals. Thirdly, to improve the quality of data collected, a new computer software system was designed for data entry with manuals defining variables to be collected. Fourthly, A new patient registration form was designed, piloted in all three hospitals and changed to suit the information needs of each hospital. Fifthly, capacity of all level of staff was developed in a series of consultative workshops on data collection, entry, analysis and use of data in patient care, reports and planning. Table 20.1 shows the various capacity building workshops and monitoring meetings . Finally, to increase capacity in the records departments, new staff were hired by two of the hospitals and National Service personnel were deployed. The new system was allowed to run for a full year while being monitored regularly.

Table 20.1: Capacity building and monitoring workshops

Number	Category and title	Participants
5	Training Workshops; **ICD- 10 Classification Training** **MHIS and ICD- 10 training** **MHIS data entry training** **Indicators in mental health and use of data in planning, management, policy planning and education;** **Report of Analysis of MHIS data**	 Prescribers/records staff/ managers of hospital Prescribers, records staff Records staff Managers/ward in-charges/ prescribers Managers/prescribers
6	Feedback meetings	Records staff, heads of departments/ wards/ managers, prescribers, data entry staff
1	Retreat	Hospital Directors, Administrators, Deputy Directors of Nurses Services/
13 13 10	Monitoring visits	Accra Psychiatric Hospital Pantang Psychiatric Hospital Ankaful Psychiatric Hospital

Equipment: Each hospital was provided with two desk-top computers with protection from electricity fluctuations, an external hard drive, a case of writable CDs, printed manuals on how to fill in registration forms, registration forms, abridged versions of the ICD-10 chapter 5 for prescribers and a summary sheet of diagnostic categories for records staff. Software was specially designed for patient data input and had an Access base front-end data entry with SQL post grid database. Work is on going to integrate this into the Ghana Health Service web-based District Health Information System which was recently deployed in all 170 districts of Ghana.

Results of intervention

A range of changes were identified in our monitoring reports and from written reports by medical students of the University of Ghana Medical School who evaluated the MHIS pre- and post-intervention, as part of the senior clerkship in Psychiatry in 2009 and 2010. Their key findings are set out in Table 20.2.

Table 20.2: Overview of MHIS in Ghana before and after intervention

	Prior to intervention	Post intervention
Legislative framework for HMIS	This comprises two Acts and a legislative instrument (LI 1628, Act 535 and Archives Administration Act 1997). governing the confidentiality of patient information, the usage, storage and handling of patient information	Remained the same.
MHIS at the psychiatric hospitals	Almost entirely paper based, with all data aggregated before entry into database. Data thus inflexible for wide range of analysis.	Individual records could be printed out and data analysis possible on wide range of variables. However, the format required demographic data to be re-entered on each visit, increasing workload of staff
Diagnostic categories:	No standardized categorization of illness within and across the three hospitals.	Use of ICD-10 R major categories for mental and behavioural disorders. Expansion of categories increased from 4 to 10

Table continued from page 259.

	Prior to intervention	**Post intervention**
Personnel:	Little allocation of resources to records departments, little training for records personnel, and with the exception of diploma level biostatisticians (one at each hospital), staff had few computer skills	Two diploma statisticians were temporarily hired by hospitals, and four polytechnic level Statistics National Service personnel were transferred to the records departments of two hospitals. Capacity of records staff was enhanced through numerous workshops and feedback meetings
Equipment and protection of data	There was one aging computer in each department, with no antivirus protection.	Better equipped records departments and computer security policy adopted.

Influencing factors

The project team reflected on the key facilitators and challenges faced. Four facilitating factors and five challenges were identified as follows.

First among the facilitators, the extensive nature of consultations with all levels of staff throughout the year of intervention ensured that mistakes of implementation were kept to a minimum. Secondly, endorsement and ownership of the project by the medical directors of the three hospitals encouraged staff to take the project seriously. Thirdly, the provision of needed logistic and financial support for the records departments helped accomplish the setting up of the MHIS. Lastly, capacity building of all relevant staff (prescribers, ward staff, records staff) was important and providing incentives for data entry by staff ensured the timeliness of data entry during the project.

The five challenges were: workload, registration form flow through the hospital, system security, capacity and sustainability. First, running two systems of MHIS was necessary for security and a check on the system but it increased workload, and staff needed constant reminding about the purpose of the new MHIS. The bi-monthly feedback of patient information to prescribers, nurses and records staff helped to maintain interest and an incentive system was put in place to motivate data entry staff but hospitals will need to motivate staff to continue this. Secondly, ensuring the smooth flow of the registration form throughout the hospital was difficult and was the subject of consultative meetings because of hospital concerns of confidentiality of patient data, and ensuring that patients would hand in the registration form at the end of the outpatient visit. Thirdly, MHAPP supplied registration forms until the hospitals were supposed to take over this task. It was difficult because of budgetary constraints and challenged the sustainability of the project. Fourthly, there was poor internet connectivity in two hospitals and therefore no easy way to update their antivirus programmesand thus protect their data. With the advent of modems, it is hoped that hospitals will equip their records departments. Fifth was the need to retain the capacity developed over the year through continuous education and feedback of results to staff.

Conclusion

Developing the MHIS led to standardization of diagnoses across three hospitals, strengthened capacity in records departments for data entry and storage, the use of data as basis for clinical and management decision-making in the three hospitals. We believe that the challenges only served to enhance the MHIS because it forced the team to find solutions and to be more collaborative.

The main lesson learned was that constant consultation made for very good progress during the year. Another lesson learned is that staff were ready to use timely MHIS generated data to enhance patient care and hospital management.

Way forward

The next step of this study is to work with the hospitals to ensure that the MHIS in the hospitals is compatible with the District Health Information Management system DHIMS and that it actually runs efficiently with outputs which are useful for planning, budgeting, etc. After that, it would be important to broaden the MHIS to the districts and regions in a manner tied to the Distrit Health Information Management System (DHIMS), so that data gathered will be national in nature and will be available for use by all health care providers in it Ghana. In the meantime, it will be useful to study factors that enhance or limit uptake of technology in MHIS in order to avoid the pitfalls of introducing more transparent systems which challenge the status quo.

References

Doku, V., Ofori-Atta, A., Akpalu, B. Osei A., Ae-Ngibise K., Awenva D., Read U., Lund C., Flisher A., Petersen I., Bhana A., Bird P., Drew N., Faydi E., Funk M., Green A., & Omar M. (2008). *A Situation Analysis of Mental Health Policy Development and Implementation in Ghana*: Mental Health and Poverty Project. Available at: http://workhorse.pry.uct.ac.za:8080/MHAPP.

Gladwin, J., Dixon, R. A. and Wilson, T. D. (2003). Implementing a new health management information system in Uganda *Health Policy and Planning* 18 (2):214-224.

Husein K., Adeyi O., Bryant, J. & Cara N. (1993). Developing a primary health care management information system that supports the pursuit of equity, effectiveness and affordability. *Social Science and Medicine* 36 (5):585-59.

Kustner, B. M., Varo, C. R. and Gonzales, F. T. (2002). The goals and method of the Andalusian case register for schizophrenia *International Journal of Social Psychiatry* 48 (1):47-57.

Odhiambo-Otieno, G. W. (2005a). Evaluation criteria for District Health Management Information Systems: Lessons from the Ministry of Health, Kenya. *International Journal of Medical Informatics* 74:31-38.

Odhiambo-Otieno, G. W. (2005b). Evaluation of existing District Health Management Information Systems: A case study of the District Health Systems in Kenya. *International Journal of Medical Informatics* 74:733-744.

WHO (2005). Mental Health Information Systems module. Mental Health Policy and Service Guidance Package. Geneva: WHO.

Chapter 21

The Way Forward for Mental Health in the 21st Century in Ghana

A. Ofori-Atta and S. Ohene

Whither goeth the field of mental health? In May 2012, the Mental Health Act was signed into Law by the President of the Republic of Ghana. It was the first legal reform in mental health since the 1970s when the law had been changed by a military fiat (NRCD 1972). The basis of the 2012 Mental Health Act (Act 865) is respect for the rights of people living with mental illness. The law makes community mental health services a priority. It also specifies the institutions and rules which will govern policy and services for mental health, including a Mental Health Authority. The Authority will have overall oversight of mental health and will collaborate with the GHS in the provision of primary mental health in general hospitals and health centres.

The way forward in mental health care provision is, therefore, a focus on different models of community care and modernization of institutional care. This is a departure from the focus on the overcrowded state psychiatric hospitals of today. There will probably be a tighter rein on the work of traditional faith healers as the Ministry of Health strengthens its regulatory responsibilities. After all, the Mental Health law states that one cannot keep a person against his will in a place not certified by the Authority for longer than 72 hours. The implication of this is that prayer camps and traditional faith healers will need to be certified to keep the mentally ill. For this to happen, the Authority will need to make explicit some minimal standards of care or guidelines by which it can certify informal community care services. As well, traditional healers and prayer camp staff will need to be taught the basics of mental hygiene and first aid for mental illness to help in the management of restless patients. This interface between the traditional beliefs of illness and the science of psychiatry and psychology will be exciting for researchers, especially in psychology and anthropology in the coming years.

Because the GHS is still responsible for primary mental healthcare, it will hire psychologists for all its regional hospitals first, as it has already begun to do, and then will hire for district hospitals. As the numbers of medical assistants in psychiatry (MAP) increase, they will have more oversight of health centres and psychiatry wings in regional and district hospitals. We foresee some clinical and counselling psychologists crossing over into psychiatry through the MAP programme if the curriculum is adjusted to encourage this high-level human resource into the field following a similar British model (Roberts, 2011). Primary health care providers such as medical assistants, psychiatric nurses and medical officers will play an increasingly greater role in the provision of mental health care as task shifting affords specialists the possibility of training other professionals to do their work under supervision. The concept of task shifting will further be broadened to use new graduates in clinical and community psychology to work alongside community psychiatry nurses within communities to improve access to psycho-education and support from a hitherto untapped resource. After all, four years of studying psychology, with some training in the management of anxiety and supportive therapy for patients in crisis would enable graduates to partner community psychiatric nurses and medical assistants in psychiatry in bringing relief and psycho-education to troubled patients within the community. We will simply call this new cadre of mental health personnel Psychcorps.

Recently, the WHO outdoored standard treatment mental health care packages for use in primary health care dubbed the MHGAP packages of care. Hopefully this will give a feeling of competence to the community care nurses and physicians who have to implement these. MHGAP may be used as a great teaching and learning tool, as well as a set of criteria to ensure quality of care. Regarding research, it enables us to test the effects of treatment, given well-defined criteria and thus provides measures against which to gauge outcome of treatment. When patients with mental illness can be treated within their communities by health care staff who also see to pregnant women and children and who are comfortable discussing treatment outcomes with them, then hopefully, this would significantly reduce the stigma associated with mental illness. We can therefore see this as the next step in community mental health care: the use of MHGAP in all primary care settings, and therefore it may be the first task of the Authority when it is set up, to train primary care staff in MHGAP.

What will all this mean to academia? With respect to medical students, we will have to find more settings within which to train them in psychiatry for two reasons; first, our current sites are overcrowded due to increasing student numbers and secondly, it makes sense to train them in primary health care settings since most of them will work in those settings and this is where most Ghanaians will first access primary mental health services. It will be important to have psychiatrists and psychologists in regional and district hospitals there to help with training, and to rotate students through posts with experienced community psychiatric nurses to improve their knowledge in community care. The current practice of rotating psychology MPhil graduate students through the teaching hospital has obviously yielded positive results in terms of practical experience for trainees, and access to supervised services for patients (See Anang et al., and Osae-Larbi et al., this volume).

Since this model works, teaching and regional hospitals will do well to hire psychologists to improve the mental health of patients. In this regard, we foresee psychologists hired through departments of psychiatry such as ours for departments of non-communicable disease such as the Sickle Cell Clinic, Department of Nuclear Medicine, HIV clinics, Diabetes and pediatric clinics. Secondly, with respect to academia, our medical schools need to reassess their human resource and infrastructure needs. It is time to be bold about building adequate structures for increased student numbers, and then to cap the numbers. It is not possible to keep increasing student numbers with the same staffing levels and same sized hospitals and expect great doctors as they qualify. And when they qualify, it may be too much to expect them to want to specialize in mental health if the current infrastructure is not overhauled and psychiatric wings provided in general hospital settings where they can liaise with their peers in other specialities for the ultimate good of the patients and for the satisfaction that comes with working with a team that thinks of health as both physical and mental. For this to happen, there is a pressing need to hire more members of faculty for psychiatry and clinical psychology. This will make it possible to practice an apprenticeship model in teaching, clinical work and research. If the focus is on community care provision, then we could begin a line of research into the most efficacious models of care within our cultural setting.

We hope that this collection of work showcases the broad scope of what we do in the Department of Psychiatry and keeps alive your interest in mental health teaching, research and care.

References

Belkin, G.S., Unützer, J., Kessler, R.C., Verdeli, H., Raviola, G. J., Sachs, K., Oswald, C., Eustache, E. (2011). Scaling up for the "bottom billion": "5 x 5" implementation of community mental health care in low-income regions. *Psychiatr Serv.* 62 (12):1494-502.

Mental Health Act 2012. (Act 846) Avaiable at: http://www.thekintampoproject.org/storage/Mental%20Health%20Act%20846%20of%202012.pdf.

Mental Health Act 1972 (NRCD 30). Available at:http://ghanalegal.com/?id=3&grp=6&t=ghana-laws

Roberts, M.(2011). Perse com on the Kintampo programme for Medical Assistants in Psychiatry programme.

WHO (2008). Mental Health Gap Action Programme : scaling up care for mental, neurological and substance use disorders.

Index

D

E

R

S

Printed in the United States
By Bookmasters